Clinical Decisions in Medically Complex Dental Patients, Part II

Editors

MEL MUPPARAPU
ANDRES PINTO

DENTAL CLINICS OF NORTH AMERICA

www.dental.theclinics.com

October 2023 • Volume 67 • Number 4

ELSEVIER

1600 John F. Kennedy Boulevard • Suite 1800 • Philadelphia, Pennsylvania, 19103-2899

http://www.dental.theclinics.com

DENTAL CLINICS OF NORTH AMERICA Volume 67, Number 4
October 2023 ISSN 0011-8532, ISBN: 978-0-323-93923-2

Editor: John Vassallo; j.vassallo@elsevier.com
Developmental Editor: Akshay Samson

Dental Clinics of North America (ISSN 0011-8532) is published quarterly by Elsevier Inc., 360 Park Avenue South, New York, NY 10010-1710. Months of issue are January, April, July, and October. Business and Editorial Offices: 1600 John F. Kennedy Boulevard, Suite 1800, Philadelphia, PA 19103-2899. Periodicals postage paid at New York, NY and additional mailing offices. Subscription prices are $333.00 per year (domestic individuals), $692.00 per year (domestic institutions), $100.00 per year (domestic students/residents), $388.00 per year (Canadian individuals), $897.00 per year (Canadian institutions), $100.00 per year (Canadian students/residents) $454.00 per year (international individuals), $897.00 per year (international institutions), and $200.00 per year (international students/residents). International air speed delivery is included in all *Clinics* subscription prices. All prices are subject to change without notice. **POSTMASTER:** Send address changes to *Dental Clinics of North America*, Elsevier Health Sciences Division, Subscription Customer Service, 3251 Riverport Lane, Maryland Heights, MO 63043. **Customer Service (orders, claims, online, change of address): Elsevier Health Sciences Division, Subscription Customer Service, 3251 Riverport Lane, Maryland Heights, MO 63043. Tel: 1-800-654-2452 (U.S. and Canada). Fax: 314-447-8029. E-mail: journalscustomerservice-usa@elsevier.com (for print support); journalsonlinesupport-usa@elsevier.com (for online support).**

Reprints. For copies of 100 or more, of articles in this publication, please contact the Commercial Reprints Department, Elsevier Inc., 360 Park Avenue South, New York, NY 10010-1710. Tel.: 212-633-3874; Fax: 212-633-3820; E-mail: reprints@elsevier.com.

The Dental Clinics of North America is covered in *MEDLINE/PubMed (Index Medicus), Current Contents/Clinical Medicine, ISI/BIOMED* and *Clinahl*.

Contributors

EDITORS

MEL MUPPARAPU, DMD, MDS
Diplomate, American Board of Oral and Maxillofacial Radiology; Professor and Director of Radiology, Department of Oral Medicine, University of Pennsylvania School of Dental Medicine, Philadelphia, Pennsylvania, USA

ANDRES PINTO, DMD, MPH, MBA, MSCE
Professor and Chair, Oral and Maxillofacial Medicine, Associate Dean for Graduate Studies, School of Dental Medicine, Case Western Reserve University, University Hospitals Cleveland Medical Center, Cleveland, Ohio, USA

AUTHORS

SUNDAY AKINTOYE, BDS, DDS, MS
Associate Professor, Department of Oral Medicine, University of Pennsylvania School of Dental Medicine, Philadelphia, Pennsylvania, USA

EMAN ALAMODI, BDS
Department of Oral Medicine, University of Pennsylvania School of Dental Medicine, Philadelphia, Pennsylvania, USA

SARA N. ALDOSARY, BDS
Department of Oral Medicine, University of Pennsylvania School of Dental Medicine, Philadelphia, Pennsylvania, USA

FATMAH ALHENDI, BMedSc, DDS, MSOB
Ministry of Health, AlSulaibikhat, Kuwait

ANGELA M. BARNES, RDH, PHDHP, MEd
Community College of Philadelphia, Philadelphia, Pennsylvania, USA

ELIZABETH BORTELL, DDS
Director of Pediatric Dentistry, Children's Hospital of Richmond at VCU, Assistant Professor, Department of Pediatric Dentistry, Virginia Commonwealth University School of Dentistry, Richmond, Virginia, USA

STEFANIA BRAZZOLI, DDS, MS
Orofacial Pain Fellow, Division of Orofacial Pain, Department of Oral and Maxillofacial Pain, Thomas Jefferson University Hospital, Philadelphia, Pennsylvania, USA

MILDA CHMIELIAUSKAITE, DMD, MPH
Assistant Professor, School of Dental Medicine, Graduate Program Director in Oral Medicine, University of Washington School of Dentistry, Seattle, Washington, USA

ADEYINKA F. DAYO, BDS, DMD, MS
Assistant Professor, Department of Oral Medicine, University of Pennsylvania School of Dental Medicine, Philadelphia, Pennsylvania, USA

PETER W. DUDA, DMD
Associate Professor, Department of Diagnostic Sciences, Rutgers University School of Dental Medicine, Newark, New Jersey, USA

KATHERINE FRANCE, DMD, MBE
Assistant Professor, Department of Oral Medicine, University of Pennsylvania School of Dental Medicine, Philadelphia, Pennsylvania, USA

MARIE D. GROSH, DNP, APRN-CNP, LNHA
Instructor, Case Western Reserve University, Frances Payne Bolton School of Nursing, Cleveland, Ohio, USA

BRAD M. HONG, BA
Research Associate, Department of Oral Medicine, University of Pennsylvania School of Dental Medicine, Philadelphia, Pennsylvania, USA

WALTER W. HONG, MD
Diplomate, American Board of Psychiatry and Neurology; Executive Director, Replimune, Clinical Development, Woburn, Massachusetts, USA

JAYAKUMAR JAYARAMAN, BDS, MDS, MS, PhD
Associate Professor, Department of Pediatric Dentistry, Virginia Commonwealth University School of Dentistry, Richmond, Virginia, USA

IRENE H. KIM, DMD, MPH
Clinical Professor, Department of Oral Medicine, University of Pennsylvania School of Dental Medicine, Philadelphia, Pennsylvania, USA

ROOPALI KULKARNI, DMD, MPH
Assistant Professor, Department of Oral Medicine, University of Pennsylvania School of Dental Medicine, Philadelphia, Pennsylvania, USA

JOEL LAUDENBACH, DMD
Diplomate, American Board of Oral Medicine; Associate Professor, Oral Medicine, Atrium Health, Oral Medicine and Maxillofacial Surgery, Charlotte, North Carolina, USA

LAUREN LEVI, DMD, MS
Clinical Assistant Professor, Division of Orofacial Pain, Department of Oral and Maxillofacial Pain, Thomas Jefferson University Hospital, Philadelphia, Pennsylvania, USA

ROGAN MAGEE, MD, PhD
Resident, Department of Neurology, Penn Medicine, Philadelphia, Pennsylvania, USA

SAHAR MIRFARSI, DDS
Diplomate, American Board of Oral Medicine; Assistant Professor, Co-Coordinator of Advanced Oral Diagnosis Workgroup, College of Dental Medicine, Western University of Health Sciences, Pomona, California, USA

PAYAM MIRFENDERESKI, DDS
Chief Resident, Department of Oral Medicine, University of Pennsylvania School of Dental Medicine, Philadelphia, Pennsylvania, USA

ARCHANA MUPPARAPU, BS
Temple University School of Medicine, Philadelphia, Pennsylvania, USA

MEL MUPPARAPU, DMD, MDS
Diplomate, American Board of Oral and Maxillofacial Radiology; Professor and Director of Radiology, Department of Oral Medicine, University of Pennsylvania School of Dental Medicine, Philadelphia, Pennsylvania, USA

SOPHIA OAK, BS
Doctoral Student, Temple University Kornberg School of Dentistry, Philadelphia, Pennsylvania, USA

PURVI C. PATEL, DMD
New York University College of Dentistry, New York, New York, USA

ANDRES PINTO, DMD, MPH, MBA, MSCE
Professor and Chair, Oral and Maxillofacial Medicine, Associate Dean for Graduate Studies, School of Dental Medicine, Case Western Reserve University, University Hospitals Cleveland Medical Center, Cleveland, Ohio

ALICIA RISNER-BAUMAN, DDS, DABSCD
Assistant Professor, Clinical Oral Medicine and Clinical Restorative Dentistry, Associate Director, Care Center for Persons with Disabilities, Department of Oral Medicine, University of Pennsylvania School of Dental Medicine, Philadelphia, Pennsylvania, USA

MIRIAM R. ROBBINS, DDS, MS, DABSCD
Professor, Clinical Oral Medicine and Clinical Restorative Dentistry, Director, Care Center for Persons with Disabilities, Department of Oral Medicine, University of Pennsylvania School of Dental Medicine, Philadelphia, Pennsylvania, USA

AIRANI SATHANANTHAN, MD
Professor of Internal Medicine, College of Osteopathic Medicine of the Pacific, Western University of Health Sciences, Pomona, California, USA

DALIA SELEEM, DDS, PhD
Assistant Professor, Acting Assistant Dean for Biomedical Sciences Curriculum, College of Dental Medicine, Western University of Health Sciences, Pomona, California, USA

RABIE SHANTI, DMD, MD
Associate Professor, University of Rutgers School of Dental Medicine, Newark, New Jersey, USA

STEVEN R. SINGER, DDS
Professor and Chair, Department of Diagnostic Sciences, Interim Director, Division of Oral and Maxillofacial Radiology, Rutgers School of Dental Medicine, Newark, New Jersey, USA

MARLIND ALAN STILES, DMD
Director, Division of Orofacial Pain, Department of Oral and Maxillofacial Pain, Thomas Jefferson University Hospital, Philadelphia, Pennsylvania, USA

ALI SYED, BDS, MHA, MS
Assistant Professor, Case Western Reserve University, School of Dental Medicine, Cleveland, Ohio, USA

TAKAKO I. TANAKA, DDS, FDS RCSEd
Professor of Clinical Oral Medicine, Department of Oral Medicine, University of Pennsylvania School of Dental Medicine, Philadelphia, Pennsylvania, USA

JACOB W. TROTTER, MD
Resident, Department of Radiation Oncology, Penn Medicine, Philadelphia, Pennsylvania, USA

LAUREN WILSON, MSN, CRNP
Nurse Practitioner, Division of Gastroenterology, Hospital of the University of Pennsylvania, Center for Inflammatory Bowel Disease, Philadelphia, Pennsylvania, USA

JANA N. YABLONSKI, RDH
Department of Oral Medicine, University of Pennsylvania School of Dental Medicine, Philadelphia, Pennsylvania, USA

Contents

Preface: Clinical Decisions in Medically Complex Dental Patients, Part II xix

Mel Mupparapu and Andres Pinto

A Patient with a History of Right-Sided Stroke and Hemiplegia, in a Wheelchair, Presents with a Complaint of Upper Left Tooth Pain 561

Miriam R. Robbins and Alicia Risner-Bauman

Patients with a history of stroke often present with numerous neurologic deficits and varying degrees of disability. Ambulation problems requiring the use of a wheelchair can make accessing and receiving dental care difficult for these patients. Side effects from medications can compromise their oral health and complicate care. Possible dexterity limitations decrease their ability to maintain their oral health. Innovative care plans and adaptations may be needed to accommodate the needs of these patients but care generally can be provided safely and effectively in the outpatient dental setting.

Nonverbal Patient with Autistic Spectrum Disorder Presents for an Initial Dental Visit 565

Alicia Risner-Bauman and Miriam R. Robbins

Autistic spectrum disorder (ASD) can be characterized by communication and social interaction difficulties, focused or repetitive behaviors, and an apathetic demeanor. The understanding level of an individual who cannot communicate cannot be assessed; therefore, we cannot assume the level of understanding of some individuals with ASD. Unfortunately, general anesthesia (GA) is oftentimes used for individuals with ASD due to their inability to cooperate, possible aggressive behaviors, and inadvertent movements, without first trying less-restrictive techniques. Teaching dentists how to develop and execute management plans without GA can increase access to dental care for this population and improve their overall health.

Patient with a History of Down Syndrome Presents for Periodic Examination and Cleaning 569

Alicia Risner-Bauman and Miriam R. Robbins

Genetic disorders such as Trisomy 21, Down Syndrome, can have numerous signs and symptoms leading to treatment complications of varying degrees. Obtaining the details regarding the patient's presentation of such disorders in addition to a thorough medical history before first seeing the patient is imperative. Treating the individual is less intimidating when you evaluate how each element affects the treatment you plan to provide and allows you to be adequately prepared to provide dental care and develop an oral health plan.

A Patient with Dementia Presents from a Nursing Home with a History of Decreased Oral Intake, Malodor, and Weight Loss 573

Miriam R. Robbins and Alicia Risner-Bauman

Individuals with dementia can present with varying challenges depending on their state of disease. The individuals caring for them may be faced with resistant behaviors when trying to provide adequate oral care. A poor oral condition can lead to decreased caloric and fluid intake causing multiple comorbidities to be exasperated due to the declining oral condition. Creating a management plan and an oral disease prevention plan are key to improving the overall health outcomes of these patients.

A Patient with Cerebral Palsy Presents for Evaluation of Third Molar Pain 577

Alicia Risner-Bauman and Miriam R. Robbins

Cerebral palsy (CP) is a developmental disorder caused by brain trauma in utero or within the first few days of life, although symptoms may not develop until early infancy. Each of the 4 types of CP has its own signs and symptoms and can present unique challenges to accessing and providing dental care. Providers may be reluctant to treat these individuals due to uncontrolled body movements, primitive reflexes, varying mental capabilities, seizures, visual and hearing impairments, dysphagia, and dysarthria.

Dental Considerations and Precautions Associated with Oral Excisional Biopsy on a Patient with Cushing's Syndrome (Hypercortisolism) 581

Sahar Mirfarsi, Dalia Seleem, and Airani Sathananthan

Chronic exposure to endogenous and exogenous glucocorticoids will cause CS. Endogenous CS is uncommon, with an annual incidence of 0.2-5 individuals per million. Endogenous causes could be 1. adrenocorticotropic hormone (ACTH) dependent or 2. ACTH independent. The use of exogenous glucocorticoids to manage chronic autoimmune or inflammatory diseases is the most common cause of CS and results in iatrogenic CS. Cushing disease is caused by excess ACTH production by a pituitary tumor. CS's clinical manifestations in the head and neck region include a moon-shaped face, acne flares, and hirsutism.

A Patient with Addison Disease (Primary Adrenal Insufficiency) Presenting for Surgical Extraction of Third Molars 585

Sahar Mirfarsi, Dalia Seleem, and Airani Sathananthan

The local prevalence of primary adrenal insufficiency (PAI) depends on various factors such as genetics, environment, and timely disease diagnosis. PAI is uncommon, and the prevalence is reported to be 2 per 10,000 population. PAI is commonly caused by an autoimmune process that destroys the adrenal gland, resulting in the loss of glucocorticoid and mineralocorticoid secretion from the adrenal cortex. The lack of cortisol results in impaired glucose/fat/protein metabolism, hypotension, increased adrenocorticotropic hormone secretion, impaired fluid excretion, and hyperpigmentation. PAI has a female predominance and is commonly seen in ages 20 to 50 years but can occur at any age.

Impacted Wisdom Teeth Removal on a Patient with Primary Hypothyroidism (Hashimoto Disease) 589

Sahar Mirfarsi and Airani Sathananthan

Thyroid gland dysfunctions can adversely affect patients' systemic health and well-being. Thyroid disease is the most common endocrine disorder. Recognizing early signs and symptoms of hypothyroidism is crucial in the early diagnosis of hypothyroidism. Oral health care providers must obtain comprehensive medical records from patients with hypothyroidism before dental treatments.

Implant Placement in a Patient with Thyromegaly Associated with Graves Disease 593

Sahar Mirfarsi, Airani Sathananthan, and Joel Laudenbach

Oral health care providers should obtain comprehensive medical records from patients with hyperthyroidism before dental treatments. Graves disease is the most common cause of hyperthyroidism. Untreated hyperthyroidism can lead to dangerous adverse effects, such as coma or death. Recognizing early signs and symptoms of hyperthyroidism is crucial in reducing complications.

Mandibular Jaw Lesion Excisional Biopsy on a Patient with Hyperparathyroidism (Primary) 597

Sahar Mirfarsi, Dalia Seleem, and Airani Sathananthan

Most of the primary hyperparathyroidism is due to adenomas in the parathyroid glands. Hypercalcemia is more common in primary hyperparathyroidism. Hyperparathyroidism may be asymptomatic and detected incidentally as part of a routine serological evaluation. Oral health care providers should recognize distinct changes in the jawbone associated with primary and secondary hyperparathyroidism.

A Patient with Hypothyroidism in Need of Periodontal Connective Tissue Graft Surgery 601

Sara N. Aldosary, Payam Mirfendereski, and Mel Mupparapu

Hypothyroidism is a condition characterized by thyroid hormone deficiency and can be caused by a variety of factors. Untreated or chronic hypothyroidism can present in adult patients as myxedema, which is characterized by symptoms including fatigue, generalized slower metabolism, weight gain, depressed mood, dry skin, and brittle hair. Hypothyroidism can have various oral manifestations, particularly in children, in whom it can delay the eruption of the dentition. Dental management of patients with hypothyroidism depends on the etiology and status of the disease and requires the consideration of other organ systems affected.

The Patient Faints in the Waiting Area with a Suspected Hypoglycemic Event 605

Milda Chmieliauskaite, Marie D. Grosh, Ali Syed, and Andres Pinto

An older adult with diabetes is taking glipizide, a sulfonylurea class drug. Subsequently, she experiences a hypoglycemic episode in the dental office. Prompt recognition of hypoglycemia and administration of glucose or sugar is vital. Patient and provider education about the risks of hypoglycemia in older adults may help to prevent future hypoglycemic episodes.

An Elderly Patient with Undiagnosed Type 2 Diabetes Mellitus Presenting for an Emergency Extraction 609

Milda Chmieliauskaite, Marie D. Grosh, Ali Syed, and Andres Pinto

In this case a patient has multiple risk factors for diabetes including periodontal disease, family history positive for diabetes, and body mass index of 24 in an Asian American. He has no medical or dental home and upon presenting to the dental office would be a good candidate for diabetes screening.

A Diabetic Patient with a Recent History of Flap and Osseous Surgery Presents Back with Bleeding and Infection 613

Milda Chmieliauskaite, Marie D. Grosh, Ali Syed, and Andres Pinto

A patient with type II diabetes and renal disease developed infection and bleeding after periodontal osseous surgery. The clinician did not adequately assess the patient's long-term glycemic status or stage of chronic kidney disease (CKD) before initiating osseous surgery. Preoperative assessment of patients with diabetes should include at a minimum an Hba1c within 3 months and estimated glomerular filtration rate for CKD.

Patient with Type I Diabetes Mellitus Develops Post-Operative Hyperglycemia After Osseous Surgery 617

Milda Chmieliauskaite, Marie D. Grosh, Ali Syed, and Andres Pinto

A patient with type I diabetes withheld her diabetes medications without consulting her physician and was not able to resume her normal diet after extensive dental surgery resulting in hyperglycemia postoperatively. Clear communication between clinicians and patient about the expected postoperative course and changes to factors that may influence glycemic control could prevent hyperglycemia in the postoperative period.

A Diabetic Patient with Acute Osteomyelitis Presenting with Jaw Pain and Submandibular Swelling 621

Mel Mupparapu, Angela M. Barnes, Archana Mupparapu, and Steven R. Singer

This case scenario shows the value of applying relevant imaging and the selection of appropriate antibiotic via culture and sensitivity before prescribing especially when dealing with a patient with type 1 Diabetes Mellitus. When confronted with a diagnosis of acute osteomyelitis, it is always better to refer the patient to a hospital for admission where the management and any other intervention is easily accomplished. Admission to the hospital, culture and sensitivity, and appropriate intravenous antibiotics may have limited the progress of the infection and ultimately may have prevented the sequestration in this patient, limiting the degree of morbidity. Monitoring and control of blood glucose levels is an important part of the management in a patient from this scenario.

A Patient with a History of Multiple Myeloma Presents for the Evaluation of Oral Lesion and Burning Sensation of the Mouth **657**

Irene H. Kim, Walter W. Hong, Sophia Oak, Brad M. Hong, and Mel Mupparapu

Multiple myeloma (MM) is a hematologic malignancy belonging to a class of disorders known as plasma cell dyscrasias. Common oral manifestations of MM include osteolytic lesions in the mandible and maxilla that can present as painful bony swellings, epulis formation, or sudden teeth movement. MM treatment is coordinated by a multidisciplinary team and is dependent upon the age and physical fitness of the patient, as well as the staging of the disease. A large proportion will be treated with intravenous bisphosphonates, such as pamidronate and zoledronic acid, which places the patients at high risk for developing medication-related osteonecrosis of the jaw (MRONJ).

A Patient Undergoing Treatment of Hematologic Malignancy Reports for Oral Evaluation **663**

Payam Mirfendereski and Katherine France

Oral lesions are commonly seen in patients with acute myeloid leukemia (AML) and may be the first clinical signs of disease. It is important for the dental provider to be able to recognize the oral manifestations of AML to allow for timely referral to a medical specialist. Patients with AML may receive treatment through chemotherapy, targeted drug therapies, or stem cell transplantation, which can involve oral complications and therefore necessitate case-specific patient education, dental evaluation, and treatment planning.

A Patient Presenting for Dental Extraction After Completion of Chemotherapy **667**

Walter W. Hong, Irene H. Kim, Brad M. Hong, Sophia Oak, and Mel Mupparapu

Acute myeloid leukemia (AML) presents several oral manifestations, including gingival hyperplasia, pale mucosa, poor wound healing, petechiae, ecchymoses, candidiasis, recurrent herpes infection, and ulcerations in the oral mucosa. Chemotherapy is the first-line treatment of AML. Common dental complications of chemotherapy include mucositis, infections secondary to profound bone marrow aplasia, and gingival bleeding. When treating patients with AML, preparing a comprehensive treatment plan is essential to help minimize their risks for developing these oral complications.

A 65-Year-Old Man with Recent History of Radiation Therapy to the Head and Neck Reporting for Treatment of a Non-restorable Tooth **671**

Payam Mirfendereski, Jacob W. Trotter, and Katherine France

Patients with a history of head and neck radiation involving or adjacent to tooth-bearing areas are at increased risk of developing osteonecrosis following dental procedures. The dental provider should thus aim to preserve the patient's dentition after radiation therapy. Root canal therapy with coronectomy may be an option for a nonrestorable tooth, whereas atraumatic extraction can be considered if retaining the tooth is impossible. When treating a patient with a history of head and neck radiation, it is recommended that the dental provider reviews the patient's radiation records and consults with the patient's radiation oncologist to better stratify treatment risks.

A Patient with a History of Tonsillar Cancer Presents for Evaluation of Exposed Alveolar Bone in the Mouth **675**

Takako I. Tanaka and Rabie Shanti

Osteoradionecrosis (ORN) is a rare but serious late complication of head and neck radiation therapy. The mandible, proximity of the primary tumor to the jawbones, radiation dose, poor oral hygiene, and smoking history are risk factors of ORN. ORN manifests as a chronic infection with exposed jawbone, which typically occurs in the first 3 years after radiotherapy; however, the risk for ORN development occurring in the patients who have undergone head and neck radiation therapy may be indefinite. Surgery has an important role in the management of cases of ORN, ranging from sequestrectomy, debridement, and extensive extirpative procedures with reconstructive surgery.

A Patient Presents for Dental Extraction and Goes into Sickle Cell Crisis in the Dental Chair **679**

Walter W. Hong, Irene H. Kim, Adeyinka F. Dayo, and Mel Mupparapu

Sickle Cell Disease is an inherited autosomal recessive hemoglobinopathy associated with multiorgan damage. This single gene disorder involves one DNA base pair alteration, producing HbS. The sickle-shaped cells form when deoxygenated in the capillaries. The resulting RBC stasis leads to ischemia and pain, and acute and chronic organ damage. Patients with SCD presenting to a dental office need careful examination to rule out any current infections, neurologic deficits, or other organ involvement before formulating a dental treatment plan to avoid prolonged and complicated procedures. Early intervention and dental anxiety management are key to the dental treatment of patients with SCD

A Patient with Refractory Trigeminal Neuralgia was Referred for Suspected Odontogenic Pain **683**

Stefania Brazzoli, Lauren Levi, Marlind Alan Stiles, and Andres Pinto

Chronic pain of the face with a sudden, unilateral, and electric shock-like pain in the distribution of the trigeminal nerve is known as Trigeminal neuralgia (TN). This case report presents a patient with TN symptoms, along with concomitant tooth pain. The diagnostic process and management of the patient are discussed, emphasizing the importance of interdisciplinary collaboration for optimal patient care.

A Patient with Herpes Zoster of the Maxillary Division of Trigeminal Nerve Presents for Oral Evaluation and Toothache **687**

Irene H. Kim, Archana Mupparapu, Jana N. Yablonski, and Mel Mupparapu

Herpes zoster (HZ) is an acute and painful neurocutaneous infection caused by the reactivation of a latent varicella-zoster virus in the dorsal root or cranial nerve ganglia. It is characterized by 3 stages: prodromal, acute, and chronic. During the prodromal stage, reactivation in the maxillary branch of the trigeminal nerve closely mimics odontalgia, and HZ should be in the differential diagnosis. Patients with HZ develop painful lesions following the affected dermatome. Laboratory testing confirms the diagnosis; treatment is with antiviral agents. Early detection and treatment shorten the course of the infection and lessen the severity of the associated postherpetic neuralgia.

Child Patient with a History of Status Epilepticus Referred for Management of Grossly Decayed Primary Molar **691**

Elizabeth Bortell and Jayakumar Jayaraman

A patient with status epilepticus presents with a grossly carious primary molar. Medical consultation is requested from the patient's neurologist. The patient is treated in the operating room under general anesthesia for comprehensive dental care.

Patient with Crohn's Disease Presents for Pain in Relation to Maxillary Teeth **695**

Payam Mirfendereski, Lauren Wilson, and Katherine France

Crohn's disease has been associated with poor oral health and oral health–related quality of life. Myriad-specific and nonspecific oral lesions have been associated with Crohn's disease. Oral lesions in patients with Crohn's disease may be a source of referred pain, especially if mucosal ulcerations or orofacial granulomatosis are involved. The dental provider can play an important role in evaluating for and/or managing oral lesions in patients with Crohn's disease and thereby improving patients' oral health and quality of life.

A Patient Diagnosed with Bulimia Reports to the Dental Office Seeking Cosmetic Dental Work **699**

Irene H. Kim, Walter W. Hong, and Mel Mupparapu

Bulimia nervosa (BN) is a serious psychiatric illness that typically occurs in adolescents and young adults. It is characterized by recurring episodes of consuming large amounts of food with an inappropriate compensatory behavior of purging to prevent weight gain. The purging behavior results in oral manifestations such as dental erosion, dental caries, sialadenosis, and oral mucosal trauma. Medical complications include electrolyte imbalances, esophageal rupture, and renal and cardiovascular failure. Treatment of BN involves psychosocial and psychopharmacologic approaches. Dentists are in a unique position to recognize patients with BN and help patients with BN and other eating disorders.

A Pregnant Patient (First Trimester) Reporting for Pain in Relation to the Maxillary Left First Molar Was Prescribed a Full Mouth Series Radiographs in the Dental Office **703**

Peter W. Duda, Steven R. Singer, Eman Alamodi, and Mel Mupparapu

This case scenario shows the value of conducting a thorough clinical examination that will direct appropriate radiographic selection and prescription criteria to be able to arrive at a diagnosis. Proper management of a patient's chief complaint and imaging needs during pregnancy is of utmost importance. It is prudent to limit ionizing radiation during the first trimester to what is minimally needed and defer elective imaging until after the birth of the baby. It is important for dental health care providers to do what is necessary for the patient for the emergent situation and postpone all elective imaging and follow the published FDA/ADA radiographic selection criteria.

A Pregnant Patient with Gestational Diabetes Reports for Scaling and Root Planning **707**

Milda Chmieliauskaite, Marie D. Grosh, Ali Syed, and Andres Pinto

In this case a woman with gestational diabetes and otherwise healthy pregnancy needs scaling and root planning for the treatment of stage I periodontal disease during pregnancy. Her daily blood sugars are in the target range, and there are no contraindications to providing necessary dental treatment under local anesthesia with vasoconstrictors in her case.

Restorative Dental Treatment and Endodontic Surgery in a Pregnant Patient Receiving Corticosteroids **711**

Fatmah Alhendi

Corticosteroid therapy (CST) can be used to treat complicated pregnancy. Second trimester of pregnancy is the preferred period to perform dental treatments. The long-term use of CST may result in hyperglycemia, hypertension, immunosuppression, and adrenal suppression, which, theoretically, may cause adrenal crisis during surgical procedures. The risk of adrenal crisis at the dental clinic caused by exogenous CST depends on the dosage, duration of treatment, route of administration, frequency, time lapse since the last dose, and type of procedure performed. Current evidence found that patients on CST undergoing general dental procedures or minor surgical procedures under local anesthesia do not require supplementary corticosteroids.

DENTAL CLINICS OF NORTH AMERICA

FORTHCOMING ISSUES

January 2024
Controversial Topics in Dentistry and Oral and Maxillofacial Surgery
Harry Dym, *Editor*

April 2024
Diagnostic Imaging of the Teeth and Jaws
Galal Omami, *Editor*

July 2024
Dental Sleep Medicine
Leopoldo P. Correa, *Editor*

RECENT ISSUES

July 2023
Clinical Decisions in Medically Complex Dental Patients, Part I
Mel Mupparapu and Andres Pinto, *Editors*

April 2023
Temporomandibular Disorders: The Current Perspective
Davis C. Thomas and Steven R. Singer, *Editors*

January 2023
Orofacial Pain Case Histories with Literature Reviews
David A. Keith, Michael E. Schatman, Ronald J. Kulich, and Steven J. Scrivani, *Editors*

SERIES OF RELATED INTEREST

Atlas of the Oral and Maxillofacial Surgery Clinics
https://www.oralmaxsurgeryatlas.theclinics.com/

Oral and Maxillofacial Surgery Clinics
https://www.oralmaxsurgery.theclinics.com/

Preface
Clinical Decisions in Medically Complex Dental Patients, Part II

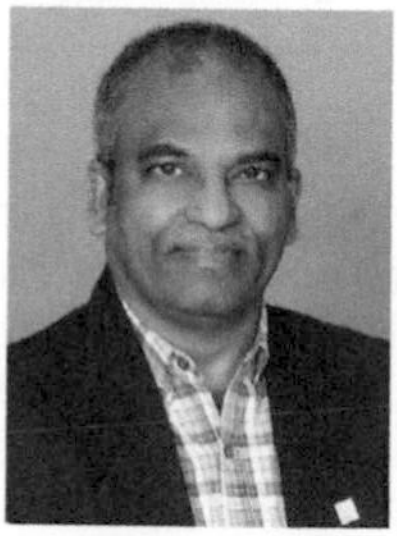

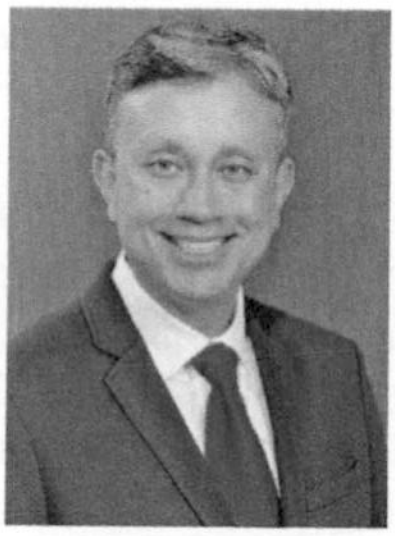

Mel Mupparapu, DMD, MDS   Andres Pinto, DMD, MPH, MBA, MSCE
Editors

After completing many scenarios in Part I of the Clinical Decisions series, like allergic reactions, anaphylaxis, renal and hepatic disorders, cardiometabolic disorders, blood dyscrasias, cerebrovascular events, and stem cell transplantation, to name a few, it is only logical in Part II to move on to other frequently encountered medical disorders that dental patients present with. If a dental practitioner is not prepared to handle a medically complex scenario, a dental practice decision and patients' well-being are in jeopardy. This *Dental Clinics of North America* Clinical Decisions Series brings to the table significant medical case scenarios and their dental chairside management of disorders such as endocrine abnormalities, autoimmune disorders, inflammatory disorders affecting bone such as osteomyelitis, challenging disorders presented by special needs patients, chronic neurologic disorders such as trigeminal neuralgia, dental treatment after chemotherapy and radiation therapy, disorders affecting the temporomandibular joints, and management of dental patients who are pregnant.

Several diseases, like multiple myeloma, sickle cell disease, Sjogren syndrome, and bulimia, that are stable after initial management but have management complexities in a dental chair are also covered in this issue. Between these two *Dental Clinics of North America* series with a focus on medical complexities and dental management decisions, we tried to present scenarios that may be noted more frequently than some. While it is difficult to cover the entirety of the medical complexities that a dental patient brings to the chair in just two issues, there are several close scenarios that very well fit the overall category of another medical complexity to arrive at a dental management decision. The practitioner can take the cues from a similar scenario.

Medical knowledge is vast and ever-changing, and we aim to have these series up-to-date for managing dental patients and act as a quick chairside reference during the dental procedure decision making.

Dent Clin N Am 67 (2023) xix–xx
https://doi.org/10.1016/j.cden.2023.05.033

As before, we used generic names for medications so that audiences worldwide may understand them without worrying about trade names. To have continuity, each case has keywords, key points, a synopsis, a medical scenario, a dental management decision with justification, and clinical care points. We used the universal tooth-numbering system in the scenarios for ease of understanding without going to the quadrant level. This continued formatting helps the clinician understand the material in a more organized manner.

We would like to thank all our authors and their families for having taken the time to contribute to this *Dental Clinics of North America* issue. We again thank our families for their encouragement and support, as we took the time away from them for editing this issue.

We thank Elsevier, publishers of the *Dental Clinics of North America*, for their help in bringing this issue in a format we thought would best serve dental practitioners, medical students, dental students, and residents. Again, we would like to thank John Vassallo, the associate publisher of the *Dental Clinics of North America*, for his encouragement and approval of this format that emerged as two issues with individualized medically complex scenarios and related dental management decisions. We would like to thank Anngie Posedio, developmental editor for Reed Elsevier, who helped us with Part I and passed the baton to Akshay Samson, our new developmental editor. Akshay did a fantastic job getting Part II together. Once again, the production team's hard work plays a crucial role in publishing the issue. We thank the data administrators and the production team specialists for their help in ensuring the material is cohesive and accurate.

The actual beneficiaries of information in the two issues are the students, residents, private practitioners, and medical and dental specialists who are in the "trenches" daily. These clinical scenarios and decisions will help them to be more attentive to their patients and be their advocates. We dedicate this issue to those busy clinicians who go beyond in the care of our patients. "May the force be with them."

Mel Mupparapu, DMD, MDS, Dipl. ABOMR
Department of Oral Medicine
Penn Dental Medicine
240 South 40th Street
Philadelphia, PA 19104, USA

Andres Pinto, DMD, MPH, MBA, MSCE
School of Dental Medicine
Case Western Reserve University
Health Education Campus
9601 Chester Avenue
Cleveland, OH 44106, USA

E-mail addresses:
mmd@upenn.edu (M. Mupparapu)
andres.pinto@case.edu (A. Pinto)

A Patient with a History of Right-Sided Stroke and Hemiplegia, in a Wheelchair, Presents with a Complaint of Upper Left Tooth Pain

Miriam R. Robbins, DDS, MS, DABSCD*,
Alicia Risner-Bauman, DDS, DABSCD

KEYWORDS

• Wheelchair • Hemiplegia • Dental care with stroke • Oral care adaptations

KEY POINTS

- Treating dental patients in wheelchairs.
- Poststroke dental needs assessment and treatment.
- Patient assessment and accommodations in poststroke patients.

SCENARIO

A 40-year-old man reports with sharp upper left tooth pain that is worse with chewing and cold that has been getting progressively worse during the previous week and now requires pain relief medication when it flares up.

Medical History

Patient had a right-sided stroke 3 years ago secondary to underlying atrial fibrillation resulting in left-sided hemiplegia. He is currently taking apixaban, metoprolol succinate, lisinopril, atorvastatin, and fluoxetine. Vital signs today are 130/84 mmHg, pulse 84. He is awake, alert, and oriented to person, place, and time with minor delay in decision-making abilities but able to provide consent for self.

Dental History

Sporadic dental care for last 3 years because of the provider's inability to accommodate a wheelchair. Third molars were extracted more than 10 years ago. Restorations

Department of Oral Medicine, University of Pennsylvania, School of Dental Medicine, 240 South 40th Street, Philadelphia, PA 19104, USA
* Corresponding author.
E-mail address: mrrobb@upenn.edu

Dent Clin N Am 67 (2023) 561–564
https://doi.org/10.1016/j.cden.2023.05.001 dental.theclinics.com
0011-8532/23/

are present. Mild-to-moderate generalized cervical plaque and calculus with increased amounts on the right maxillary posterior and lower lingual anterior areas with moderate gingival inflammation. Moderate xerostomia secondary to medication. Buccal cervical caries noted #12, 13, and 15. Bite wing radiographs more than 2 years ago. Uses manual toothbrush 2 times per day with fluoride toothpaste and is not able to floss since stroke because of manual dexterity limitations.

Social History

Patient uses motorized wheelchair for ambulation and prefers to remain in chair for treatment. Reports living at home with parents since the stroke, previously lived independently. Works part time substitute teacher.

DENTAL MANAGEMENT DECISION AND JUSTIFICATION

Comprehensive history obtained before patient arrival. Because the patient does not transfer, the wheelchair was backed against the dental chair and the headrest reversed to provide support. Full mouth radiographs and comprehensive examination were completed. Cold testing and evaluation of occlusion determined reversible pulpitis secondary to buccal caries on upper second molar as the source of discomfort. Two carpules of 2% lidocaine with 1:100,000 epinephrine delivered via infiltration was used. Caries excavation revealed deep caries without pulp exposure. A restoration was placed following an indirect pulp cap. Patient tolerated care without complications. A preventive plan including oral hygiene instruction with adaptive toothbrush and introduction of mechanical toothbrush and oral irrigation flosser, 1.1% neutral sodium fluoride toothpaste prescribed bid, and prophylaxis with 3-month recall interval and fluoride varnish application was formulated.

Accommodating patients with wheelchairs depends on several factors: approximate size of the chair, whether the chair can recline, office size and layout, and whether the user can transfer or uses a Hoyer lift.[1,2] If you do not have a Hoyer lift, the patient needs to be informed before their arrival so they can plan appropriately for toileting needs, long-term chair use, and so forth. Wheelchair tilt devices are available but the cost balanced against the amount of use and room to use may not be feasible for most practitioners. In addition to backing the patient to the dental chair, support boards and pillows can be placed between the patient and their chair[2] to provide proper head support.

Specific neurologic deficits that may be present secondary to stroke present treatment challenges for the patient and the provider (**Table 1**).[3] Addressing the oral health of these patients is critical to their overall health and preventing the worsening of comorbidities that may have led to the ischemic event.[4] This critical role of the dental provider in the recovery of these patients should be focused on disease prevention and early treatment interventions. Orofacial and tongue paralysis can lead to an increased accumulation of food debris on the affected side. Impaired dexterity, especially if on the dominant side, can decrease the patient's ability to provide effective oral hygiene. Oral health professionals need to assess the patient's abilities and teach them how to accommodate limitations to aid in their own oral care. The prevention plan developed needs to be reassessed at each recall visit, and more frequent recall may be necessary.[5]

Modifications to treatment should be based on the degree of neurologic impairment and any underlying comorbidities. Mouth props can be used during treatment if patients have difficult remaining open due to muscle dysfunction. Vital signs should be monitored at every visit. Local anesthetics with vasoconstrictors limited to 2 carpules

Table 1
Neurologic deficits secondary to ischemic stroke

Neurologic Deficits and Disability	Oral Health Management
Hemiparesis/hemiplegia	Modify oral care implements, monitor breathing, teach care givers, accommodate positioning with pillows, and other support
Cognitive deficits	Consent issues, understanding and following instructions
Hemianopia	Inability to see mouth, demonstrations, read clearly
Aphasia	Need to develop communication, longer appointments
Sensory deficits	Need to accommodate for office and home care
Depression	Medications can cause xerostomia, may not be motivated for self-care
Leg and ambulation impairment	Accommodate wheelchair or other mobility devices
Bladder incontinence	Numerous breaks, time and location to change incontinence items
Dysphagia	Airway protection, altered diet can lead to oral disease
Visuospatial neglect	Adaptive equipment for oral health
Arm and hand impairment	Adaptive equipment for oral health, assistance with home care

Many observed 6 mo postevent.[1]

should be used to ensure profound anesthesia. All oral antithrombotic medications should be continued even for surgical procedures and local hemostatic measures used to ensure good bleeding control as needed.

CLINICS CARE POINTS

- It is important to assess the patient's medical and physical condition before providing dental treatment. This includes a review of their medical history, current medications, and any physical limitations related to their wheelchair use.
- Vital signs should be monitored at every visit.
- Local anesthetics with vasoconstrictors limited to 2 carpules should be used to ensure profound anesthesia.
- All oral antithrombotic medications should be continued with the use of local hemostatic measures to help control bleeding as needed.
  Dental care should be focused on disease prevention and early treatment interventions
  Modifications to treatment should be based on the degree of neurologic impairment and any underlying comorbidities
- Consider the patient's comfort during treatment, including the use of cushions or supports to alleviate pressure on the back and legs.
- Communication with the patient should consider any hearing or vision impairments that they may have.

DISCLOSURE

The authors have no financial or other interests to disclose.

REFERENCES

1. Rashid-Kandvani F, Nicolau B, Bedos C. Access to Dental Services for People Using a Wheelchair. Am J Public Health 2015;105(11):2312–7.
2. Ramirez L, Dickinson C. Wheelchair users: a guide. BDJ Team 2018;5:18074.
3. Overview of ischemic stroke prognosis in adults. Literature review by Edwardson, M. UpToDate. Topic 14086 Version 24.0 Available at: https://www.uptodate.com/contents/overview-of-ischemic-stroke-prognosis-in-adults. Accessed Aug 15, 2022.
4. Institute of Medicine (US) Board on Health Care Services. The U.S. Oral health workforce in the coming decade: workshop summary. Washington (DC): National Academies Press (US); 2009. p. 2. The Connection Between Oral Health and Overall Health and Well-Being. Available at: https://www.ncbi.nlm.nih.gov/books/NBK219661.
5. Singh N. Treating dental patients with special needs and complex medical histories. Decisions in Dentistry 2019;5(5):30–2, 35.

Nonverbal Patient with Autistic Spectrum Disorder Presents for an Initial Dental Visit

Alicia Risner-Bauman, DDS, DABSCD*,
Miriam R. Robbins, DDS, MS, DABSCD

KEYWORDS

- Autism • Dental • Nonverbal • Behavior management • Prevention

KEY POINTS

- Preappointment assessment provides the outline for a successful first dental visit.
- Behavior modification plans need to be personalized and evolving.
- Preventive dental care can prevent overutilization of general anesthesia in patients with autistic spectrum disorder.

MEDICAL SCENARIO

A 23-year-old male patient with autistic spectrum disorder (ASD) presents for an initial dental visit.[1] A comprehensive medical, dental, and behavioral history (hx) was obtained before the patient first presented at the dental office. His mother stated that she has problems with helping her son brush his teeth because he bites on the toothbrush. She notices that his gums bleed when she can brush his teeth.

Medical hx is significant for ASD and he takes melatonin 10 mg at bedtime, risperidone 1.0 mg/d. All his immunizations are current.

Dental treatment (tx) has been under general anesthesia (GA) every 3 years. At his last operating room (OR) visit, a comprehensive examination with a full mouth set of radiographs and a full mouth scaling and root planning were completed. Three third molars were extracted, and 3 composite restorations to treat Class II D2 caries were completed.

His mother is his legal guardian. He is nonverbal. Patient (Pt.) tends bite wrist when he gets frustrated. He eats a regular consistency diet but has many food aversions. He lives at home and can perform most ADLs with minimal supervision. His mother accompanies him to his appointments and must have a driver with her so that she can supervise him.

Department of Oral Medicine, University of Pennsylvania, School of Dental Medicine, 240 South 40th Street 215, Philadelphia, PA 19104, USA
* Corresponding author.
E-mail address: arbdds65@upenn.edu

Dent Clin N Am 67 (2023) 565–568
https://doi.org/10.1016/j.cden.2023.05.002

Pt. will brush his own teeth. His mother supervises, and then she tries to brush again. He bites on the toothbrush preventing her from being able to do a thorough job. She is not able to floss.

DENTAL MANAGEMENT AND DECISION JUSTIFICATION

Obtaining a thorough history and disease risk assessment is a key first step in treating an individual with ASD because symptoms will vary for every individual. Comorbidities, dental tx. history, sensory limitations, and challenges to oral care at home will provide insight into accommodations that will increase the likelihood of a successful first visit.[2] Individuals with ASD oftentimes are taking medications with side effects that influence their oral health such as xerostomia, increasing their caries risk; dysphagia, increasing their aspiration risk; dysgeusia, leading to poor dietary choices; and gingivitis, causing increased periodontal destruction.[2] The history above reveals a patient who can be taught self-care, who needs supervision in public, and has some aversion to oral care at home done by another individual. He will hurt himself but there is no report of aggression toward others. He has a high disease risk based on his earlier treatment needs. Prevention of oral disease is paramount in keeping this patient out of the OR and will be the most important part of this patient's overall dental treatment plan, such as 3-month recall visits with fluoride varnish applications. Addressing the global challenges individuals with ASD face including food aversions, lack of cooperation, self-injurious behaviors, and communication challenges in a personalized prevention plan is important to maintaining their overall health.[3]

Treatment without GA will require patience and time. Successful treatments can be achieved by developing an evolving treatment-modification plan using manageable goals for each visit based on the patient's response to care at each visit (**Box 1**). Desensitization, such as allowing the patient to wander the operatory and office to become familiar with the dental environment, is often successful because routine and familiarity are considered key treatment interventions for individuals with ASD.[4] Teaching this mother how to use a mouth prop during oral care because he bites the toothbrush is a good first-visit goal that with direct oversight will allow a provider

Box 1
Behavior management techniques to use for patients with complex medical or behavioral histories that require extra time, staff, and/or expertise in order to receive services

- *Complex medical*: Several comorbidities, numerous medications to monitor, physically limiting conditions, compromised airway, positioning restrictions.
- *Tell-show-do*: Tell what you are going to do; show what you are using, allow to touch, hear, and so forth; and then do procedure, after clearing that they understand if possible to evaluate.
- *Positive reinforcement*: A behavior is followed by the presentation of an appetitive (desired) stimulus, increasing the probability of that behavior.
- *Communicate with the patient*: Discuss problems and solutions and what you are doing whether or not they can respond or are "capable" of understanding. Communicate to the patient's intellectual level. Storyboards can be used to share ideas and communicate expectations.
- *Shaping by successive approximations*: A behavioral method that reinforces responses that successively approximate and ultimately match the desired response.
- *Distractions:* Using the environment to redirect the patient's attention from procedure.

- *Desensitization*: Dividing procedures into pieces and conquering each one separately. Methodical introduction of stimuli to accomplish final goal.
- *Determined technique*: Count and break technique in which set amount time will be used for procedure; patient is then given a break. Patient is informed of how much time they must cooperate, what going to do during that time, and told that they will be given a break at that time (counting up to 5, gradually increasing to 10, and so forth).

Developed by Dr David Tesini, available from Specialized Care Company, http://www.specializedcare.com.

- *Modeling*: Showing what doing in different setting or on different subject.
- *Decision-making*: The process of choosing between alternatives; selecting or rejecting available options. Choices should be limited; choices should not include doing desired actions.
- *Perceived control*: The thought that one has the ability to make a difference in the course or the consequences of some event or experience; often helpful in dealing with stressors. Giving control back to the patient over what their fear or anxiety factors may be.
- *Limiting movements*: Limiting movements that prevent interference with care and holds of short duration for safety.
  - *Medical immobilization and/or protective stabilization*: Manual, physical, or pharmacologic limitation of unfavorable actions.
  - Definitions provided by Glossary of Psychological Terms from American Psychological Association http://www.apa.org/research/action/glossary.aspx?tab=18

A specific plan should be developed for each individual. Use the least restrictive method needed to accomplish task. Record amount of time needed, number of staff required if over and above norm for procedure, specific behavior being managed, techniques tried in the past, medical and behavioral history, and action plan to decrease need. No Creditline.

to do a screening examination of the patient. Introducing items to be used at the next visit should be sent home with instructions on use for desensitization, such plastic mirrors, disposable prophy angles, and x-ray sensor holders, for example. More involved procedures can be introduced once a patient learns the routine of the office, has a consistent provider and staff, and is allowed to progress at their own pace.[2] Management of disease prevention and behavioral challenges is paramount in creating a dental home for individuals with ASD.

CLINICS CARE POINTS

- Obtaining a thorough medical, dental, and behavioral history before first clinic visit allows practitioners to be prepared to accommodate the individual's needs before their arrival providing a smoother introduction to the new environment and people.[2]
- Maintaining oral health in this population can require the involvement of the individual and the caregivers. Providing instructions to both improves health outcomes for this population.[3]
- Nonrestrictive techniques can be successfully used to treat patients with ASD when oral care providers are patient and willing to learn these techniques, thus reducing the number of cases referred for treatment with GA and decreasing the risks associated with GA when treating this population.[5]

DISCLOSURE

The authors have no financial or other interests to disclose.

REFERENCES

1. Goldstein G, Allen D, Deluca J. 4th edition. Handbook of psychological assessment. Amsterdam: Academic Press; 2019.
2. Chandrashekhar S, S Bommangoudar J. Management of autistic patients in dental office: a clinical update. Int J Clin Pediatr Dent 2018;11(3):219–27.
3. Schmalz G, Ziebolz D. Changing the focus to the whole patient instead of one oral disease: the concept of individualized prevention. Advances in Preventive Medicine 2020;1–11. https://doi.org/10.1155/2020/6752342.
4. Health, N. I. (2022). Autism Spectrum Disorder. Retrieved from National Institute of Mental Health website: Available at: nimh.nih.gov/health/topics/autism-spectrum-disorders-asd. Accessed July 20, 2022.
5. Lim MAWT, Borromeo GL. The use of general anesthesia to facilitate dental treatment in adult patients with special needs. J Dent Anesth Pan Med 2017;17(2):91–103.

Patient with a History of Down Syndrome Presents for Periodic Examination and Cleaning

Alicia Risner-Bauman, DDS, DABSCD*,
Miriam R. Robbins, DDS, MS, DABSCD

KEYWORDS

• Down syndrome • Dental management • Medical management

KEY POINTS

- Understanding the various presentations of signs and symptoms of genetic disorders is necessary to accommodate the needs of individuals.
- Individuals with Trisomy 21, Down Syndrome can usually be treated in an outpatient setting.
- Management plans for individuals with Down Syndrome will be dependent upon the medical, behavioral, and dental history of the individual. Each of these aspects will require a plan to be consolidated into one general approach to care.

MEDICAL SCENARIO

A 28-yr-old patient with Down Syndrome (DS) reports for recall examination and continued preventive care (**Table 1**). Prior to the initial visit, a thorough medical, dental, and social history were obtained.

Med hx

Atrioventricular septal defect (AVSD) repaired in infancy with no residual cardiac effects; partial seizures treated with 100 mg b.i.d. Phenytoin ER (last seizure 5+ yrs. ago); mild intellectual disability (IQ ~ 65); hypothyroidism treated with 100mcg Levothyroxine/day; mild obesity (ht. 5′5″, wt. 165lbs); atlantoaxial insufficiency.

Dental hx

3 month recall interval; moderate caries risk with increased soda intake, mouth breathing and a history of Class V white lesions; good oral hygiene with light generalized cervical and moderate interproximal plaque, light calculus lower anterior teeth,

Department of Oral Medicine, University of Pennsylvania, School of Dental Medicine, 240 South 40th Street 205, Philadelphia, PA 19104, USA
* Corresponding author.
E-mail address: arbdds65@upenn.edu

Dent Clin N Am 67 (2023) 569–571
https://doi.org/10.1016/j.cden.2023.05.003
dental.theclinics.com

Table 1
Common features of down syndrome and management[1–5]

Dental/Oral	Systemic
• Midface insufficiency: difficulty breathing through nose, may require more breaks, nitrous use challenging: inc. flow • Megaglossaly: decreases airway, increases risk during treatment and sedation: HVE, RD, isolating mouth pieces • Congenitally missing secondary teeth: spacing concerns, may need to treat primary teeth for long-term function • Open bite: makes biting and chewing difficult, can inc. choking risk, inc. GI upset: orthodontic correction if oral hygiene is good • Dysphagia: increased aspiration risk HVE, RD, isolating mouth pieces • Fissured Tongue: increased bacterial load: show how to clean • Low caries rate: dependent on diet • Speech Apraxia: may require assistance to communicate • Feeding Disorders: may use GI tube or require extra feeding time: emphasize need for proper oral care despite no oral intake	• Intellectual limitation: may not understand or follow instructions: keep simple • Congenital heart condition: may require antibiotic prophylaxis • Immune suppression: may require antibiotics or miss appointments • Respiratory problems: watch positioning and have O2 available • Vision problems: may be light sensitive, allow to feel things, warn when entering mouth • Hypothyroidism: monitor HR and temp • Atlantoaxial insufficiency: provide neck support from chair or pillows • Limited dexterity: provide adaptive equipment • Gastrointestinal Disorders: improve chewing and monitor medications • Movement problems: may require stabilization: manual or mechanical with consent • Sleep Disorders: CPAP machines can dry out oral cavity: provide saliva substitutes • Seizures: type, frequency, safety measures, medications can affect oral tissues • Hearing Loss: watch for hearing aids and speak clearly

minimal inflammation, and no alveolar loss; megaglossaly; Class III malocclusion with anterior open bite; retained #a,j,k,t and missing #1,4,7,10,13,16,17,18,20,29, 32; mild speech apraxia. Cooperative for care after several desensitization appointments with this office to accommodate dental anxiety. Hx. of treatment with sedation prior to this office.

Other hx

Lives with parents who are legal guardians and supportive decision makers, has a part time job at a local store, and graduated high school. Likes to paint and shows some of his artwork at a local gallery on a regular basis.

DENTAL MANAGEMENT DECISION AND JUSTIFICATION

Patient. reports no pain or swelling currently. Recall examination with radiographs, prophylaxis, and fluoride varnish application. Radiographs are made with assistance (provider holding sensor in pt. mouth) since pt. is unable to bite the sensor holder and remain still. A supportive pillow is placed between the patient's neck and the dental chair to support the neck due to atlantoaxial insufficiency. Patient likes to hold mirror and watch procedure as well as use the saliva ejector by themselves. Patient wears their own sunglasses for visits due to light sensitivity. Patient continues to use mechanical toothbrush and high concentration fluoride toothpaste twice daily. Recommendation: To maintain 3 mo recall interval until overall hygiene has improved.

The presentation of Down syndrome will vary for individuals with unique signs and symptoms that need to be addressed to provide safe and effective care.[1,3,5] Consultations with PCPs and specialists may be needed, and interviewing care givers is imperative. As noted in **Table 1**, it is best to address each finding in the context of their influence on the treatment planned. A comprehensive management plan will include managing the oral, medical, behavioral, and social findings.[2,3,5] These plans are meant to be fluid, and should be evaluated as treatment progresses.

CLINICS CARE POINTS

- It is important to obtain a thorough medical, dental, and social history prior to the patient's arrival so that medical consultations and treatment adaptations can be completed and the first appointment dedicated to treating the patient.[1,5]
- Communicating directly with the patient regardless of intellectual limitations or ability to respond is critical to developing trust, showing empathy, and maintaining patient autonomy.[1,5]
- Patient's with Down Syndrome can present with complicating malocclusions and congenitally missing teeth that create not only dental restorative concerns but also medical management concerns. Dentists need to be familiar with the various comorbid oral conditions present in order to safely provide care to the patient with Down Syndrome.[3]

DISCLOSURE

The authors have no financial or other interests to disclose.

REFERENCES

1. Abanto J, Ciamponi AL, Francischini E, et al. Medical problems and oral care of patients with Down syndrome: a literature review. Spec Care Dentist 2011;31(6):197–203.
2. Trisomy 21 (Down Syndrome). Available at: https://www.chop.edu/conditions-diseases/trisomy-21-down-syndrome. Accessed August 25, 2022.
3. Macho V, Coelho A, Areias C, et al. Craniofacial features and specific oral characteristics of Down syndrome children. Oral Health Dent Manag 2014;13(2):408–11.
4. Down Syndrome. Available at: https://www.cdc.gov/ncbddd/birthdefects/downsyndrome.html. Accessed on August 25, 2022.
5. Intellectual Disability. Available at: https://www.psychiatry.org/patients-families/intellectual-disability. Accessed July 31, 2022.

A Patient with Dementia Presents from a Nursing Home with a History of Decreased Oral Intake, Malodor, and Weight Loss

Miriam R. Robbins, DDS, MS, DABSCD*,
Alicia Risner-Bauman, DDS, DABSCD

KEYWORDS

• Oral health • Oral hygiene • Dementia • Caries risk assessment

KEY POINTS

- Patients with dementia are at a higher risk for poor oral health due to factors such as decreased oral hygiene, impaired cognitive and physical abilities, and side effects of medications.
- The focus on dental interventions in patients with dementia should be on the prevention of dental disease and infection.
- Maintaining good oral hygiene is important to prevent dental caries, gum disease, and other oral health problems in patients with dementia.
- Caregivers should assist patients with dementia in maintaining good oral hygiene by helping them brush their teeth and assisting with denture care if needed.

SCENARIO

78-year-old presented with staff from nursing facility with consultation form requesting evaluation for limited oral intake, malodor, and weight loss. Medications and current medical diagnoses were listed on the consultation. Patient was not able to answer questions in coherent fashion, and not willing to open mouth when requested. Information obtained regarding who provides consent for care, supervising physicians, and oral care information from the long-term care facility prior to appointment.

Department of Oral Medicine, University of Pennsylvania, School of Dental Medicine, 240 South 40th Street, Room-209A, Philadelphia, PA 19104, USA
* Corresponding author.
E-mail address: mrrobb@upenn.edu

Dent Clin N Am 67 (2023) 573–576
https://doi.org/10.1016/j.cden.2023.05.004
0011-8532/23/

Medical History

Mild dehydration, recent weight loss (17lbs), hypertension, dementia, and osteoarthritis. Medications include nifedipine, hydrochlorothiazide, ramipril, donepezil. rivastigmine, trazodone, risperidone, and ibuprofen. Vital signs were 112/66, pulse of 64.

Examination was. accomplished after moisturizing lips, using spoon as prompt to open, and inserting a mouth prop. Patient was wearing a maxillary partial denture with erythema present under denture base clinically consistent with candidal infection. Examination of the dentition revealed multiple carious and fractured teeth along with moderate calculus and soft debris and gingivitis. There were no obvious swelling or signs of active odontogenic infection noted. A full mouth series of radiographs was obtained with the provider stabilizing the patient's head and sensors with mouth prop in place. The final diagnosis was generalized periodontal disease, carious teeth (some non-restorable) and denture stomatitis. Treatment plan included thorough plaque and calculus debridement with chlorhexidine rinse, smoothing of sharp cusps causing soft tissue trauma, caries control utilizing silver diamine fluoride and preventive restorations, and treatment of both oral cavity and prosthesis for candida. Non-restorable teeth were evaluated individually for signs of active infection, mobility, and need for surgical intervention vs observation.

Dental History

The patient had received regular dental care until admitted to nursing facility 4 years ago. Annual examination by facility dentist was limited due to the lack of cooperation. Patient was unable to provide own oral care. Nursing staff reported inability to provide oral care due to patient resistance including swatting, turning head, and refusal to open mouth.

DENTAL MANAGEMENT DECISION AND JUSTIFICATION

Management and treatment of a patient with dementia can be challenging depending on the stage of the dementia for not only oral health care providers, but for caregivers as well. The progression and stage of the dementia affects how the patient will cope with dental treatments and what interventions might be needed (**Box 1**). The focus of dental interventions in patients with dementia should be on the prevention of dental disease and maintenance of the best oral health possible. Because of the progressive nature of the disease, thorough oral assessment, and early intervention to improve oral health is imperative. A comprehensive extraoral and intraoral hard and soft tissue intraoral examination; appropriate radiographic examination; and evaluation of removable prostheses (if present) should be completed as part of the oral health assessment. If the patient is considered incapable of making their own medical decisions, involvement of those persons with medical power of attorney for all planning and treatment appointments is required.[1]

Behavioral management techniques can be effective in the treatment of patients with dementia. Having someone familiar to the patient in the treatment room can be beneficial. Using a calm voice, offering frequent reassurances, and minimizing external environmental stimulation and distractions can be employed. Nonverbal communication, such as sitting at the patient's level, direct eye contact and gentle contact (such as touching an arm or patting a shoulder) should also be utilized.[2] The goals of treatment planning should emphasize control of dental disease and prevention of infection and pain.[3] Caries risk assessment and use of minimally invasive dentistry should be incorporated into treatment planning.[4] Silver diamine fluoride application along with atraumatic restorative technique are essential tools in the treatment of this population.[5]

Box 1
Dental care for patients with dementia

Early-Stage Dementia
- Routine dental care with minor modifications
- Treatment plans anticipating that patient will eventually not be able to care for teeth
- All restorations easily cleansable
- Plan to "jump" fixed prosthesis to removable
- More aggressive prevention
- Stress importance of preventive oral hygiene
- Educate family member/caregiver as well
- Use electric toothbrushes and irrigation aids
- Make use of memory aids
  - Pictures, instruction lists, audio aides

Moderate-Stage Dementia
- Focus changes from restorative to prevention
- Expect resistant behavior
- May not be possible to do a thorough examination
- Shorter appointments
- Eliminate any sources of pain or potential infection
- May be able to do simple restorative
- Use alternative remineralization/caries arrest approach
- Treatment plans
  - Minimal changes
  - Reline rather than remake dentures
  - If making new dentures, use old ones to recreated overall shape and tongue space
- Caregivers responsible for OH
- Education and reinforcement

Late-Stage Dementia
- Prevention of dental disease
- Maintaining oral comfort
- Provision of emergency care
- Focus on pain/infection
- May leave root tips if non-symptomatic
- IV sedation/general anesthesia
  - Only when absolutely necessary
- Maintain dentition with frequent oral hygiene measures
  - More frequent recalls
  - Fluoride varnish every visit
- SDF and preventive restorative as needed

More frequent recare appointments with the application of fluoride varnish at each appointment can also be employed to prevent decline in the oral health.

Education of caregivers in how to deliver adequate oral hygiene is also essential. Similar to the delivery of dental care, non-pharmacologic behavior management techniques can be utilized to facilitate oral home care plan. for these individuals. These can include the use of stabilization techniques, disposable mouth props, modified oral hygiene devices, and prescription fluoride toothpastes. Chlorohexidine swabs can be used if patients are unable to swish and spit. Proper denture hygiene should also be reinforced and include removal of the prostheses after meals and before bed and proper cleaning and storage.

CLINICS CARE POINTS

- Caries risk assessment and the use of minimally invasive dentistry should be incorporated into treatment planning.

- Silver diamine fluoride used with atraumatic restorative technique are vital tools in the management of oral disease in this population
- Education of caregivers on the importance of the delivery of daily oral hygiene care is essential and should be reinforced at every visit.

DISCLOSURE

The authors have no financial or other interests to disclose.

REFERENCES

1. Fabiano JA. Oral health management in the patient with dementia. Medscape 2011;24.
2. Marchini L, Ettinger R, Caprio T, et al. Oral health care for patients with Alzheimer's disease: an update. Spec Care Dentist 2019;39:262–73.
3. Oong EM, An GK. Treatment planning considerations in older adults. Dent Clin North Am 2014;58:739–55.
4. Chavez EM, Wong LM, Subar P, et al. Dental care for geriatric and special needs populations. Dent Clin North Am 2018;62:245–67.
5. Crystal YO, Niederman R. Evidence-based dentistry update on silver diamine fluoride. Dent Clin North Am 2019;63(1):45–68.

A Patient with Cerebral Palsy Presents for Evaluation of Third Molar Pain

Alicia Risner-Bauman, DDS, DABSCD*,
Miriam R. Robbins, DDS, MS, DABSCD

KEYWORDS

• Cerebral palsy • Spasticity • Wheelchair • Oral diagnosis

KEY POINTS

- Cerebral palsy has many presentations; therefore, a proper assessment needs to be done to accommodate the needs of the individual.
- Symptoms including lack of mobility, dexterity limitations, and involuntary movements are among some of the symptoms that can limit one's ability to access oral care.
- Comorbidities can complicate the oral presentation of individuals with cerebral palsy.
- Oral health complications associated with cerebral palsy may include sialorrhea, attrition due to bruxism, muscle spasms, increased caries, and periodontal disease.

SCENARIO

A 23-year-old patient reports with "wisdom tooth" pain of 3-month duration that causes intermittent sharp discomfort.[1] A comprehensive medical, dental, and social history was obtained before the patient first presented at the dental office.

Medical History

Medical history includes the use of baclofen, 15 mg, 3 times a day for muscle spasms due to spastic cerebral palsy (CP); carbamazepine, 800 mg/day, for seizure control; omeprazole, 20 mg/day, for gastroesophageal reflux disease; senna 2 tablets/day pro re nata (PRN) constipation; and 1000 mg acetaminophen PRN pain. Depression and anxiety are not treated with medication.

Dental History

Patient has had routine recall examinations every 6 months. Last radiographs were 18 months ago. She has had intermittent treatment of parafunctional activity. She

Department of Oral Medicine, University of Pennsylvania, School of Dental Medicine, 240 South 40th Street 215, Philadelphia, PA 19104, USA
* Corresponding author.
E-mail address: arbdds65@upenn.edu

Dent Clin N Am 67 (2023) 577–579
https://doi.org/10.1016/j.cden.2023.05.023
0011-8532/23/

Table 1
Types of cerebral palsy[2]

Type	Symptoms	Management
Spastic	Increased muscle tone, contractures, described by body part affected	Need to stabilize for patient and provider safety, interferes with oral care
Dystonic/ dyskinetic	Problems controlling movements, varying muscle tome	Stabilization, inability to clear oral cavity, assistance for oral care
Ataxic	Problems with balance and coordination	Accommodate mobility devices, adaptive oral care equipment
Mixed	Combination of the aforementioned	Combination of the aforementioned

has mild sialorrhea secondary to uncoordinated swallowing (dysphagia). She uses a motorized toothbrush, an oral irrigator for interdental cleaning daily, and fluoride toothpaste without assistance.

Social History

Patient has difficulty with verbalization (dysarthria), uses crutches to aid ambulation, and lives independently. She uses her parents' insurance and discusses treatment with them although she can give consent for her own care.

DENTAL MANAGEMENT DECISION AND JUSTIFICATION

A comprehensive oral examination using a rubber mouth prop to prevent spastic closure reveals a severely worn dentition with a slight anterior open bite, bilateral muscle spasms, and white 5- to 7-mm ulcerated lesions with keratinized borders on the buccal mucosa near the second molar. A panoramic radiograph made with stabilization devices to stop involuntary movement showed no evidence of third molar development. Minimal plaque and calculus with no inflammation were seen. The mostly likely cause of the lesions noted was traumatic secondary to buccally inclined molars.

CP types, spastic, dyskinetic, ataxic, and mixed, present with varying symptoms and severity (**Table 1**). Numerous comorbidities may present themselves secondary to the severity of the disease that affect not only overall health but also the general well-being of these individuals.[2] Mouth props, stabilization, assistance with oral hygiene, and an aggressive prevention plan can improve the provider's ability to treat these individuals. A comprehensive evaluation of the patient's *abilities* needs to be made before any comprehensive oral health care can be provided.[3]

Ambulation and dexterity concerns are common for individuals with CP due to muscle dystonia and/or spasticity.[4] Patients may exhibit an exaggerated bite reflex, and

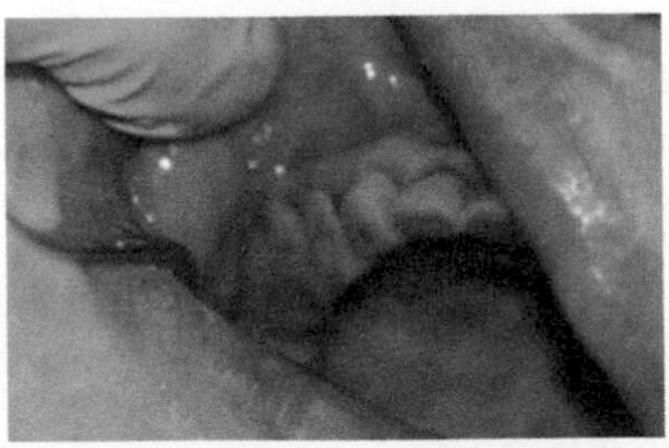

Fig. 1. Severe occlusal wear in a patient with CP. (Photo by Alicia Risner-Bauman.)

use of mouth props is warranted. Often an assisted technique is needed to stabilize the patient. Assistance may be needed to hold radiographs in place for the patient in order to get diagnostic images. To evaluate third molar pain, a panoramic film was preferred but without stabilization a diagnostic image may not have been obtained. In this case, the pain from the buccal ulcers was mistaken for "wisdom tooth" pain by the patient. Bruxism is a common finding for these individuals, sometimes leading to pulp exposure (**Fig. 1**). Careful evaluation of the dentition and soft tissues is needed, and occlusal guards or full coronal coverage may be needed if treatment can be tolerated by the individual.[3] Patients with CP often have hyperactive gag reflexes, and care should be used with suction tips and instruments not to stimulate a gag reflex. Use of digital scanning in place of traditional impressions may facilitate the fabrication of prosthetics.

CLINICS CARE POINTS

- Comprehensive oral evaluation is needed to properly diagnose pain.
- Patients can be stabilized and radiographs obtaind by using an assisted method to hold the sensor apparatus intraorally for the patient who cannot bite and hold on their own.
- Severe bruxism is a common finding in patients with cerebral palsy and they must be monitored regularly.

REFERENCES

1. Cerebral palsy. Bethesda (MD): National Library of Medicine; 2020. Available at: https://medlineplus.gov/cerebralpalsy.html. Accessed August 29, 2022.
2. Cerebral palsy in adults. London: National Institute for Health and Care Excellence (NICE); 2019 (NICE Guideline, No. 119).
3. Practical oral care for people with cerebral palsy. Bethesda (MD): National Institute of Dental and Craniofacial Research; 2009. Available at. www.nidcr.nih.gov. Accessed August 29, 2022.
4. Cerebral palsy. Rochester, (MN): Mayo Clinic; 2021. Available at. https://www.mayoclinic.org/diseases-conditions/cerebral-palsy/symptoms-causes/syc-20353999. Accessed on August 30, 2022.

Dental Considerations and Precautions Associated with Oral Excisional Biopsy on a Patient with Cushing's Syndrome (Hypercortisolism)

Sahar Mirfarsi, DDS[a,*], Dalia Seleem, DDS, PhD[a],
Airani Sathananthan, MD[b]

KEYWORDS

• Hypercortisolism • Cushing's syndrome • Adrenal crisis • Corticosteroids
• Endocrine disease

KEY POINTS

- Oral Health care providers must obtain comprehensive medical records from patients exposed to high glucocorticoid concentrations.
- Long-term exposure to exogenous glucocorticoids is the most common cause of iatrogenic CS.
- Chronic exposure to glucocorticoids in patients with CS can cause medical conditions such as hypertension, osteoporosis, and diabetes mellitus.
- Oral health care providers should carefully plan dental surgical procedures in patients with CS to avoid the risk of iatrogenic jaw fractures.

MEDICAL SCENARIO

A 54-year-old European female presented to her oral health care provider (OHCP) for the evaluation of a tender mandibular gingival mass with intermittent bleeding when flossing. The clinical exam reveals a left mandibular lobulated buccal gingival mass between teeth #19-20 (**Fig. 1**). An excisional biopsy is recommended to confirm the diagnosis. Her past medical history is significant for obesity and asthma. She has been taking systemic corticosteroids to manage her asthma frequently over the last five years. She mentions that since the Covid-19 pandemic, she has only seen her

[a] Western University of Health Sciences, College of Dental Medicine, 309 E. 2nd Street, Pomona, CA 91766, USA; [b] Western Universit of Health Sciences, Department of Internal Medicine, 795 E 2nd Street, Pomona, CA 91766, USA
* Corresponding author.
E-mail address: Sahar.mirfarsi@westernu.edu

Dent Clin N Am 67 (2023) 581–584
https://doi.org/10.1016/j.cden.2023.05.005
0011-8532/23/

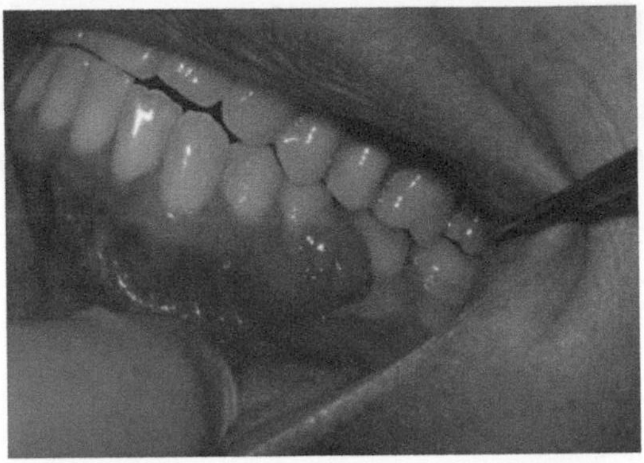

Fig. 1. Exophytic and lobulated mass on the left mandibular buccal gingiva, between teeth #20-19. An excisional biopsy and histopathology analysis confirmed the diagnosis of a peripheral ossifying fibroma. (*Courtesy of Sahar* Mirfarsi, DDS.)

primary care physician via telehealth visits. She reports increased fatigue, back pain, headaches, and generalized distal muscle weakness. In addition, she reports uncharacteristic irritability and anxiety for the last 1.5 years.

Vital Signs and Other Findings

Blood pressure: 159/93 mm Hg.

Heart rate: 75 beats per minute.

Fasting blood glucose: 189 mg/dL.

Body mass index: 42 kg/m^2.

On physical examination, she has moon facies, central obesity, and pinkish-purple striation on the arms and abdomen. In addition, she has atrophy of the skin of the arms as well as a dorsocervical fat pad. The patient was referred to her primary care physician for further evaluation of suspected Cushing's syndrome (CS).

Dental management decision and justification

Chronic exposure to endogenous and exogenous glucocorticoids will cause CS.[1] Endogenous CS is uncommon, with an annual incidence of 0.2-5 individuals per million.[2,3] Endogenous causes could be.

1. Adrenocorticotropic hormone (ACTH) dependent or
2. ACTH independent.[2]

Use of exogenous glucocorticoids to manage chronic autoimmune or inflammatory diseases is the most common cause of CS and results in iatrogenic CS.[1,3] Cushing disease is caused by excess ACTH production by a pituitary tumor.[1] CS's clinical manifestations in the head and neck region include a moon-shaped face, acne flares, and hirsutism.[1]

Early diagnosis of CS to reduce mortality from cardiovascular disease, infection, psychiatric diseases, diabetes mellitus, and osteoporosis is crucial.[3] Therefore, OHCPs should be aware of concomitant medical conditions such as hypertension, heart failure, depression, psychosis, diabetes mellitus, and osteoporosis in patients with CS due to long-standing exposure to glucocorticoids.[3]

OHCPs should consult with physicians before dental treatment in patients with CS to see if an adjustment in steroids is warranted. **Box 1** highlights some questions to consider asking physicians regarding suspected patients of CS. OHCPs should

Box 1
Medical consult questions to ask physicians regarding CS

- What are the current medications, in particular steroids? Dosages? Frequencies?
- Does the patient need prophylactic antibiotic coverage for dental procedures?
- Has the patient ever experienced an adrenal crisis?

monitor vital signs, including blood pressure at baseline and during dental appointments, to avoid severe hypertensive episodes while using epinephrine in local anesthetic. Abrupt disruption in corticosteroid use could cause the impairment of the hypothalamic-pituitary-adrenal axis and result in an adrenal crisis.[3] Adrenal crisis can present with hypotension, hyperthermia, nausea, vomiting, and abdominal pain.[1] Consulting with physicians is necessary to evaluate the need for stress dose steroids before major oral and maxillofacial surgeries.[3]

Patients undergoing moderate to high dose glucocorticoid therapy are considered immunosuppressed.[3] Therefore, OHCPs should be aware of patients developing oral candidiasis, recurrent herpes stomatitis, gingival and periodontal diseases.[3] In addition, patients with CS are susceptible to delayed wound healing and infections[4]; therefore, OCHPs should consult with the patient's physician and consider antibiotic prophylaxis before dental surgical procedures, especially in immunosuppressed patients with active dentoalveolar infections.[3]

Chronic exposure to glucocorticoids can cause osteoporosis; therefore, caution is needed to prevent iatrogenic jawbone fractures, especially during procedures with substantial mechanical manipulations.[1] Patients with CS may be at increased risk of peptic ulceration[3]; therefore, OHCPs should be cautious in prescribing postoperative analgesics such as aspirin and non-steroidal anti-inflammatory medications. In addition, certain drugs can interact with glucocorticoids, such as fluconazole, ketoconazole, and long-term use of clarithromycin.[5]

In this case, hypercortisolism was caused by prolonged and exogenous exposure to corticosteroids for asthma control. However, our patient also had an elevated fasting blood glucose; therefore, further evaluation is needed to assess the underlying diabetes mellitus. In addition, OHCPs must monitor blood pressure and glycemic control before dental procedures.

CLINICS CARE POINTS

- Obtain comprehensive medical records in patients with CS, including the dosage and frequency of glucocorticoids.
- OHCPs should avoid the abrupt discontinuation of corticosteroids and consult with the patients' physicians.
- Be aware of drug interactions with patients who are taking glucocorticoids.
- Monitor vital signs at baseline and during dental procedures to avoid hypertensive episodes.
- OHCPs should carefully evaluate pain management with aspirin and NSAIDs in patients with CS at risk of peptic ulcer.

DISCLOSURE

The authors have nothing to disclose/disclosures.

REFERENCES

1. Farag AM. Head and Neck Manifestations of Endocrine Disorders. Atlas Oral Maxillofac Surg Clin North Am 2017;25(2). https://doi.org/10.1016/j.cxom.2017.04.011.
2. Ahmed SF, Bapir R, Fattah FH, et al. Simultaneous pituitary and adrenal adenomas in a patient with non ACTH dependent Cushing syndrome; a case report with literature review. Int J Surg Case Rep 2022;94:107038.
3. Glick M, Greenberg MS, Lockhart PB, Challacombe SJ, eds Burket's Oral Medicine. Wiley; 2021. https://doi.org/10.1002/9781119597797.
4. Fabue LC, Soriano YJ, Pérez MGS. Dental management of patients with endocrine disorders. J Clin Exp Dent 2010;2(4). https://doi.org/10.4317/jced.2.e196.
5. David Erskine- Specialist Pharmacy Services (SPS), elen Simpson on behalf of Society for Endocrinology Steroid Emergency Card working group. Exogenous Steroids Treatment in Adults.

A Patient with Addison Disease (Primary Adrenal Insufficiency) Presenting for Surgical Extraction of Third Molars

Sahar Mirfarsi, DDS[a,*], Dalia Seleem, DDS, PhD[a],
Airani Sathananthan, MD[b]

KEYWORDS

- Primary adrenal insufficiency • Addison disease • Glucocorticoids
- Endocrine disease • Oral health care providers

KEY POINTS

- Endocrine dysfunctions can adversely affect the overall systemic health and well-being of patients.
- Oral health care providers should recognize primary adrenal insufficiency's unique oral mucosal and skin manifestations.
- Adrenal gland destruction due to autoimmune processes is the common cause of primary adrenal insufficiency.
- Oral health care providers must obtain comprehensive medical records from patients with Addison disease before dental treatments.

MEDICAL SCENARIO

A 45-year-old European women with a past medical history of Hashimoto thyroiditis and type 1 diabetes presented to a dental office for evaluation of mandibular third molars for surgical extraction. The patient reports a darkening of her skin and hyperpigmentation of her oral mucosa (**Figs. 1** and **2**). The review of systems is significant for dizziness, fatigue, nausea with occasional vomiting, and progressive weight loss over the last 8 months. However, she denies headaches, blurred vision, changes in bowel habits, or loss of consciousness.

---

[a] Western University of Health Sciences, College of Dental Medicine, 309 East Second Street, Pomona, CA 91766-1854, USA; [b] Western University of Health Sciences, College of Osteopathic Medicine of the Pacific, Department of Internal Medicine, 309 East Second Street, Pomona, CA 91766-1854, USA

* Corresponding author. Western University of Health Sciences, College of Dental Medicine, 309 East Second Street, Pomona, CA 91766-1854.
E-mail address: sahar.mirfarsi@westernu.edu

Dent Clin N Am 67 (2023) 585–588
https://doi.org/10.1016/j.cden.2023.05.006

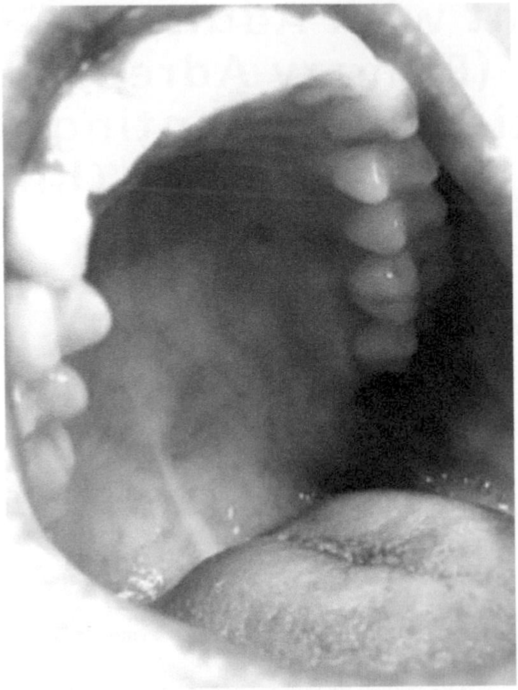

Fig. 1. Multiple irregular flat brown pigmentations on the soft palate, gingiva, and lips in a patient diagnosed with Addison disease. (*Courtesy of* Sahar Mirfarsi, DDS.)

Vital Signs and Other Findings

Blood pressure: 90/50 mm Hg.

Pulse: 75 beats per minute.

Respiration: 24 breaths per minute.

Fasting blood glucose: 65 mg/dL.

Because of her symptoms, the patient sought evaluation by her primary care provider.

Laboratory Values

Thyroid-stimulating hormone: 3.25 mU/L (normal range: 0.46–4.68 mU/L).

Morning serum cortisol level less than 3 mg/dL (8 AM normal range 5–23 mg/dL).

Hemoglobin A1C: 6.5% (diabetes goal target <7%).

Cosyntropin stimulation test results confirmed the diagnosis of Addison disease.

DENTAL MANAGEMENT DECISION AND JUSTIFICATION

The local prevalence of primary adrenal insufficiency (PAI) depends on various factors such as genetics, environment, and timely disease diagnosis.[1] PAI is uncommon, and the prevalence is reported to be 2 per 10,000 population.[2] PAI is commonly caused by an autoimmune process that destroys the adrenal gland, resulting in the loss of glucocorticoid and mineralocorticoid secretion from the adrenal cortex.[3] The lack of cortisol results in impaired glucose/fat/protein metabolism, hypotension, increased adrenocorticotropic hormone (ACTH) secretion, impaired fluid excretion, and

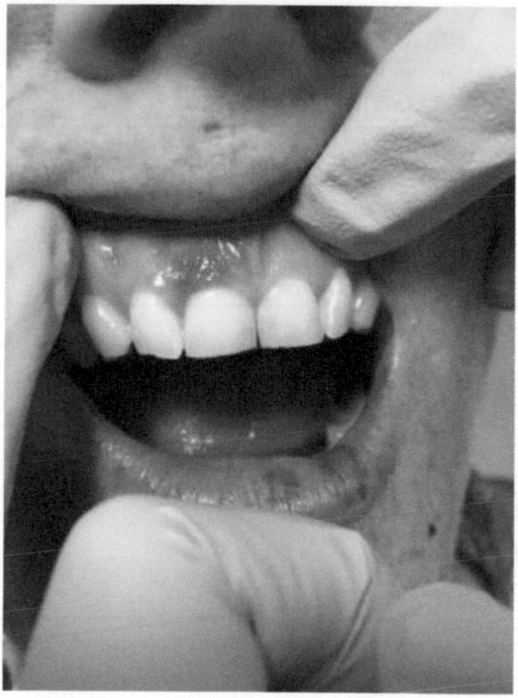

Fig. 2. Multiple irregular flat brown pigmentations on the soft palate, gingiva, and lips in a patient diagnosed with Addison disease. (*Courtesy of* Sahar Mirfarsi, DDS.)

hyperpigmentation. PAI has a female predominance and is commonly seen in ages 20 to 50 years but can occur at any age.[2]

Identifying hyperpigmentation of the skin and oral mucosal membranes should warrant further workup for this disease.[3] Low cortisol levels and loss of negative regulatory feedback on the hypothalamus and pituitary result in increased production of proopiomelanocortin, ACTH, and melanocyte-stimulating hormone, which increases melanogenesis and results in hyperpigmentation. Oral mucosal hyperpigmentation from PAI is asymptomatic. An acute adrenal crisis can result in a medical emergency at the dental office.[4] Adrenal crisis in PAI has an incidence of 5 to 10 events per 100 patients/year.[2]

Oral health care providers (OHCPs) are in a unique position to identify abnormalities associated with PAI. Stress and surgery can induce an adrenal crisis, and postural hypotension may progress to hypovolemic shock.[4] Therefore, minimizing stress during surgical procedures will reduce adrenal crisis.[3] Medical management of PAI includes glucocorticoid and mineralocorticoid replacement. Most patients with PAI may undergo routine dental treatments, including minor dental surgeries under local anesthetic, without the need for additional corticosteroid supplementation.[4] However, OHCPs should be vigilant in assessing patients' needs for stress dose steroids, especially during major surgeries requiring general anesthesia.[3,4]

Monitoring vital signs before dental procedures is essential.[4] Normally, cortisol is secreted in response to stress. In patients with PAI, cortisol production in response to stress is insufficient. As a result, patients are at increased risk of developing severe hypotension and cardiac complications such as stroke, coma, and death.[4]

The need for corticosteroid supplementation should be discussed with the patient's physician. The supplementation regimen includes doubling the daily dose of oral

Table 1
Corticosteroid supplementation recommendation in stressful events[5]

Stress Intensity	Surgical Procedure	Recommended Additional Supplementation
Mild	Minor dental surgery (eg, tooth extraction)	25 mg/day of hydrocortisone on the day of surgery
Moderate	Moderate dental surgery (eg, 2 jaw surgeries)	50–75 mg/day of hydrocortisone for 1–2 days
Severe	Major dental surgery (eg, head and neck reconstruction or resection)	100–150 mg/day of hydrocortisone for 2–3 days

corticosteroids the day before the dental surgery and the day of the dental surgery.[5] **Table 1** outlines the recommendation for steroid supplementation during surgery based on the complexity of the dental surgery. OHCPs may need to administer intramuscular or intravenous hydrocortisone in an acute adrenal crisis.[5] This case demonstrates the need to consult with the physician after evaluating the surgical stress a patient may undergo before surgical tooth extraction.

CLINICS CARE POINTS

- Obtain comprehensive medical records in patients with Addison disease, including the dosage and frequency of glucocorticoids.
- Oral mucosal hyperpigmentation may present as the initial manifestation of Addison disease.
- Monitor vital signs at baseline and during dental procedures to avoid hypotensive episodes.
- Most patients undergoing minor dental procedures with local anesthetic will not require corticosteroid supplementation.
- Stress dose steroids may be necessary before major dental surgeries requiring general anesthesia.
- OHCPs should consult with patients' physicians regarding corticosteroid supplementation.

DISCLOSURE

The authors have nothing to disclose.

REFERENCES

1. Saverino S, Falorni A. Autoimmune addison's disease. Best Pract Res Clin Endocrinol Metab 2020;34(1):101379.
2. Hahner S, Ross RJ, Arlt W, et al. Adrenal insufficiency. Nat Rev Dis Prim 2021;7(1):19.
3. Thoppay JR, Sollecito TP, De Rossi SS. Oral Signs of Endocrine and Metabolic Diseases. In: Fazel N, editor. Oral Signs of Systemic Disease. Cham: Springer; 2019. https://doi.org/10.1007/978-3-030-10863-2_4.
4. Farag AM. Head and neck manifestations of endocrine disorders. Atlas Oral Maxillofac Surg Clin North Am 2017;25(2). https://doi.org/10.1016/j.cxom.2017.04.011.
5. bin Rubaia'an MA, Alotaibi MK, Alotaibi NM, et al. Cortisol in oral and maxillofacial surgery: a double-edged sword. Int J Dent 2021;2021:1–8.

Impacted Wisdom Teeth Removal on a Patient with Primary Hypothyroidism (Hashimoto Disease)

Sahar Mirfarsi, DDS[a,*], Airani Sathananthan, MD[b]

KEYWORDS

- Hashimoto thyroiditis • Endocrine disease • Oral health care providers
- Hypothyroidism • Myxedema

KEY POINTS

- Thyroid gland dysfunctions can adversely affect patients' systemic health and well-being.
- Thyroid disease is the most common endocrine disorder.
- Recognizing early signs and symptoms of hypothyroidism is crucial in the early diagnosis of hypothyroidism.
- Oral health care providers must obtain comprehensive medical records from patients with hypothyroidism before dental treatments.

MEDICAL SCENARIO

A 39-year-old Middle Eastern woman with a history of Hashimoto thyroiditis was referred to a local oral and maxillofacial surgery office for evaluation of impacted wisdom teeth, #17 and 32, surgical extractions. She has been on variable doses of levothyroxine but a few months ago decided to discontinue to see if she had any improvement in her vertigo. She is recently experiencing increased fatigue, difficulty losing weight, occasional constipation, and cold intolerance. However, she noted no significant difference in her vertigo since stopping the levothyroxine.

Vital Signs and Other Findings

Blood pressure: 99/66 mm Hg.
Heart rate: 53 beats per/min.

[a] College of Dental Medicine, Western University of Health Sciences, 309 East 2nd Street, 3rd Floor, Pomona, CA 91766, USA; [b] College of Osteopathic Medicine of the Pacific, Western University of Health Sciences, Pomona, CA, USA
* Corresponding author. Western University of Health Sciences, College of Dental Medicine, 309 East Second Street, Pomona, CA 91766-1854.
E-mail address: Sahar.Mirfarsi@westernu.edu

Dent Clin N Am 67 (2023) 589–592
https://doi.org/10.1016/j.cden.2023.05.007

Respiratory rate: 19 breaths per/min.
Weight: 203 lbs (92.1 kg).
Body mass index: 33.78 kg/m^2.

Review of System

The patient seems overweight and not in acute distress. No thyromegaly was noted on the examination.

Laboratory Workup from the Primary Care Physician

Thyroid-stimulating hormore: 63.09 mIU/L (normal range: 0.40–4.5 mIU/L).
Free thyroxine (T4): 0.6 ng/dL (normal range: 0.8–1.8 ng/dL).
Antithyroid peroxidase antibody: 72.6 IU/mL (normal range: 0–34 IU/mL).
Fasting blood glucose: 100 mg/dL (normal range: 65–99 mg/dL).
High-density lipoprotein: 49 mg/dL (normal range: > OR = 50 mg/dL).
Low-density lipoprotein (LDL): 103 mg/dL (normal range: 99 mg/dL).

DENTAL MANAGEMENT DECISION AND JUSTIFICATION

Thyroid disease is the most common endocrine disease.[1] The thyroid hormone is essential for the growth and development of infants and children. In addition, the thyroid hormone plays a significant role in energy metabolism in adults. The hypothalamus-pituitary axis feedback mechanism is crucial in controlling the thyroid glands' function.[2] Hypothyroidism is referred to as deficiency of thyroid hormone production, low thyroxine (T4) and/or triiodothyronine (T3), that can be related to congenital defects, autoimmune disease, or acquired factors such as a history of radioactive iodine therapy or thyroidectomy.[2] Myxedema refers to skin changes in adults with long-lasting hypothyroidism.[1] In myxedema, mucopolysaccharide accumulation in the subcutaneous tissue may present as nonpitting edema in hands, feet, and eyelids.[3]

Up to 5% of the general population is affected by hypothyroidism.[1] In developed countries, chronic autoimmune thyroiditis or Hashimoto thyroiditis is the most common cause of hypothyroidism.[1] Hashimoto thyroiditis is due to high-level circulating autoantibodies against thyroid peroxidase, the necessary enzyme to convert T4 to T3.[1] Women are more affected than men.[1] Because of the high prevalence, oral health care providers (OHCPs) must recognize early signs and symptoms of hypothyroidism (**Table 1**).[4]

Patients with an autoimmune thyroid disorder (Hashimoto thyroiditis) may develop other autoimmune connective tissue disorders such as Sjögren syndrome.[5] Patients with thyroid complaining of hyposalivation and xerophthalmia should be further evaluated for possible Sjögren syndrome (**Fig. 1**). Although most patients with well-

Table 1
Mild-moderate hypothyroidism signs and symptoms[4]

Mild-moderate hypothyroidism signs and symptoms	Weight gain Fatigue Depression Menstrual irregularities Dry hair Thick and dry skin Cold intolerance Bradycardia Voice deepening

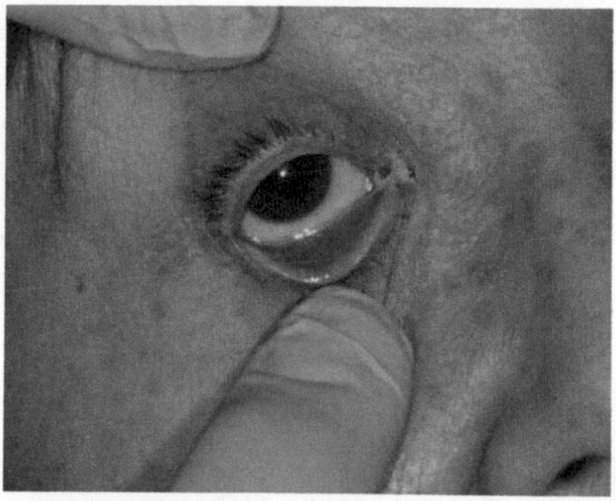

Fig. 1. Xerophthalmia in a female patient with well-controlled Hashimoto thyroiditis and a recent diagnosis of Sjögren syndrome.

controlled hypothyroidism do not require special dental precautions or modifications, it is crucial to consult with the patient's primary care physician to obtain a comprehensive general clinical history, current laboratory values, and the status of their disease before dental procedures. In addition, monitoring vital signs during dental procedures is essential to avoid complications.[4]

OHCPs should palpate the anterior neck region and feel for any swelling or goiter as part of their comprehensive oral examination at every dental visit.[3] In patients with Hashimoto thyroiditis, the thyroid gland will feel much firmer on palpation than the normal gland.[3] Sodium levothyroxine (LT4) is a synthetic preparation of thyroxine used to treat patients with hypothyroidism.[4,5] Patients with hypothyroidism are also at risk for developing atherosclerosis from cardiovascular disease and elevated LDL.[1] Patients with myxedema are at risk for developing bleeding postsurgical dental procedures due to the inability of small vessels to constrict and mucopolysaccharide infiltration of tissues, including in mucosa.[5] In addition, wound healing may be delayed due to reduced fibroblast metabolic activity.[4]

Uncontrolled hypothyroidism can lead to respiratory depression; therefore, placing patients in a partially upright position and providing oxygen supplementation may be necessary. In addition, stress during dental procedures should be minimized. If needed, prescribing medications that can induce central nervous system depression, including narcotics for postoperative pain management, should be prescribed in consultation with a physician.[4]

Epinephrine in local anesthetic or gingival retraction cords can potentially cause adverse effects with existing cardiac symptoms in uncontrolled hypothyroidism and should be used with caution.[4] Myxedematous coma is an extreme manifestation of hypothyroidism in patients with uncontrolled hypothyroidism. Signs of myxedematous coma include severe alteration of the mental status, hypothermia, arrhythmia, severe hypotension, and epileptic seizure.[4]

CLINICS CARE POINTS

- Obtain the patient's most recent medical records.
- Monitor vital signs at baseline and during dental procedures to avoid complications.

- Epinephrine in local anesthetic should be used with caution in uncontrolled hypothyroidism.
- Reduce stress during dental procedures.
- At every dental examination visit, palpate the thyroid gland to detect swelling or changes.
- Most patients with controlled disease undergoing routine dental procedures will not require modifications.

DISCLOSURE

The authors have nothing to disclose.

REFERENCES

1. Chiovato L, Magri F, Carlé A. Hypothyroidism in context: where we've been and where we're going. Adv Ther 2019;36(S2):47–58.
2. Rees TD, Endocrine and metabolic disorders. In: Patton LL, Glick M, The ADA Practical Guide to Patients with Medical Conditions. 2nd ed. Hoboken, NJ: John Wiley & Sons, Inc; 2016. 71–99. doi:10.1002/9781119121039. ch4.
3. Little JW. Thyroid disorders. Part II: hypothyroidism and thyroiditis. Oral Surg Oral Med Oral Pathol Oral Radiol Endod 2006;102(2):148–53.
4. Farag AM. Head and neck manifestations of endocrine disorders. Atlas Oral Maxillofac Surg Clin North Am 2017;25(2). https://doi.org/10.1016/j.cxom.2017.04.011.
5. Fabue LC, Soriano YJ, Pérez MGS. Dental management of patients with endocrine disorders. J Clin Exp Dent 2010;2(4). https://doi.org/10.4317/jced.2.e196.

Implant Placement in a Patient with Thyromegaly Associated with Graves Disease

Sahar Mirfarsi, DDS[a,*], Airani Sathananthan, MD[b],
Joel Laudenbach, DMD[c]

KEYWORDS

• Graves disease • Endocrine disease • Oral health care providers • Hyperthyroidism
• Goiter

KEY POINTS

- Oral health care providers should obtain comprehensive medical records from patients with hyperthyroidism before dental treatments.
- Graves disease is the most common cause of hyperthyroidism.
- Untreated hyperthyroidism can lead to dangerous adverse effects, such as coma or death.
- Recognizing early signs and symptoms of hyperthyroidism is crucial in reducing complications.

MEDICAL SCENARIO

A 33-year-old Caucasian man presented to our dental office for implant placement in the edentulous alveolar ridge of missing left mandibular first and second molars, #18 and 19. In the past 3 years, he has lost multiple teeth due to extensive caries. In addition, he reports increased hunger, a 6 to 8 lbs weight loss, palpitations, insomnia, frequent bowel movements, and heat intolerance. He had similar symptoms when he was diagnosed with hyperthyroidism about 2 years ago and took methimazole for 1 year. He went to the emergency department 1 week ago.

The Laboratory Values in the Emergency Department

Thyroid-stimulating hormone (TSH): <0.008 mIU/L (normal range: 0.550–4.780 mIU/L).
Free T4: 5.7 ng/dL (normal range: 0.89–1.70 ng/dL).

[a] College of Dental Medicine, Western University of Health Sciences, 309 East 2nd Street, 3rd Floor, Pomona, CA 91766, USA; [b] College of Osteopathic Medicine of the Pacific, Western University of Health Sciences, Pomona, CA, USA; [c] Atrium Health Oral Medicine & Maxillofacial Surgery, 1601 Abbey Place, Suite 220, Charlotte, NC 28209, USA
* Corresponding author. Western University of Health Sciences, College of Dental Medicine, 309 East Second Street, Pomona, CA 91766-1854.
E-mail address: Sahar.Mirfarsi@westernu.edu

Dent Clin N Am 67 (2023) 593–596
https://doi.org/10.1016/j.cden.2023.05.008
dental.theclinics.com
0011-8532/23/

Since the emergency department visit, he has been taking propranolol, 10 mg, every 8 hours and methimazole, 20 mg, daily with some improvement in his symptoms. On physical examination, he has thyromegaly with a thyroid bruit, mild proptosis, tremors on extension of the hands, and mild hyperreflexia.

Vital Signs

Blood pressure: 163/94 mm Hg.
Heart rate: 103 beats per/min.
Respiratory rate: 18 breaths per/min.

DENTAL MANAGEMENT DECISION AND JUSTIFICATION

Thyroid disease is a common endocrine condition. Hyperthyroidism is caused by an overactive thyroid gland, resulting in the overproduction of circulating thyroxine (T4) and triiodothyronine (T3).[1] Graves disease (diffuse toxic goiter) is the most common cause of hyperthyroidism.[2] It is an autoimmune disorder in which the thyrotropin receptor antibodies activate the TSH receptor, resulting in increased thyroid hormone synthesis and secretion.[3] Graves disease is more common in women and younger patients.[2] Exophthalmos can be associated with Graves disease.[3]

Well-controlled patients with hyperthyroidism require no special precautions.[2] However, if an undiagnosed case of Graves disease is suspected, the oral health care provider (OHCP) should obtain medical consultation from a physician before any elective dental procedures.[4] OHCPs should be vigilant regarding the signs and symptoms of hyperthyroidism. Untreated hyperthyroidism can lead to an acute life-threatening thyroid crisis, also known as a "thyroid storm," which can result in death or coma. Minimizing stress during dental procedures is important to reduce the risk of a thyroid storm.[2] Thyrotoxic crisis can follow dental surgical procedures; therefore, OHCPs need to recognize the signs and symptoms associated with a "thyroid storm" (**Table 1**).[3]

Abnormal signs and symptoms from head and neck examinations, such as dysphagia, or tongue swelling, can be valuable clues for thyroid diseases.[2,3] OHCPs should palpate the lower anterior neck region and feel for any goiter (thyroid gland enlargement) as part of their comprehensive oral examination at every dental visit. Goiter in Graves disease may feel softer than a normal gland would.[3] One of the most serious complications of Graves disease is cardiac issues.[4] OHCPs should use epinephrine in local anesthetics with caution due to the increased risk of tachycardia and dyspnea in patients with poorly controlled hyperthyroidism.[2] Patients with atrial fibrillation might be placed on anticoagulant therapy; therefore, prolonging the prothrombin time could cause excess bleeding or risk of hemorrhage during dental surgical procedures and should be taken seriously.[3] Agranulocytosis is a potential

Table 1
Thyrotoxic crisis symptoms[3]

Thyrotoxic crisis symptoms[3]	Tachycardia or arrhythmia Pulmonary edema Sweating Nausea and vomiting Fever Delirium, stupor Abdominal pain Seizure

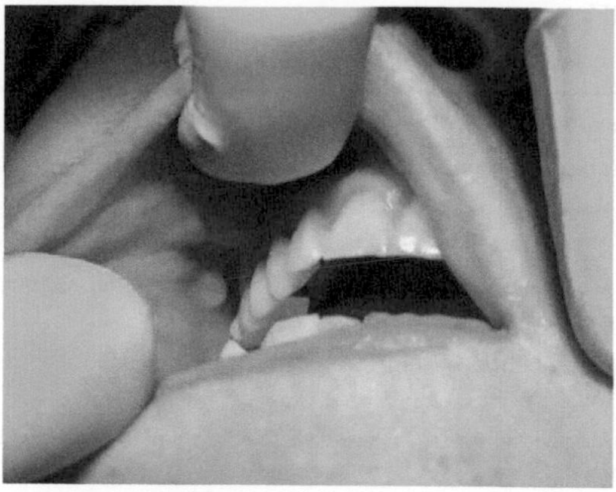

Fig. 1. Recurrent bacterial sialadenitis in a patient with a history of radioactive iodine (I-131) therapy. (*Courtesy of* Sahar Mirfarsi, DDS.)

side effect of antithyroid agents, which can increase the risk of postoperative infections.[3]

Elevated blood pressure and arteriolar pressure may increase the risk of bleeding from invasive dental procedures; therefore, extended local pressure might be necessary to stop the bleeding.[2] OHCPs should be cautious when prescribing analgesics containing acetylsalicylic acid or nonsteroidal antiinflammatory drugs (NSAIDs) due to interferences with T4 and T3 protein binding and elevation in circulating T4, causing thyrotoxicosis.[4] Patients on nonselective β-blockers for cardiovascular disease comorbidity can experience reduced effects of β-blockers while taking NSAIDs.[5] OHCP should be cautious in using epinephrine in local anesthetic or retraction cords in patients with hyperthyroidism and those taking nonselective β-blockers such as propranolol.[5]

Graves disease is often managed by radioactive iodine (RAI) therapy, thyroidectomy, or antithyroid medications such as methimazole.[1] RAI therapy can severely damage the salivary glands, especially parotid glands, resulting in chronic sialadenitis (inflammation of the salivary glands) and/or recurrent bacterial sialadenitis[1] (**Fig. 1**). Hyposalivation (**Fig. 2**) and dysgeusia can also develop in patients with a history of post-RAI therapies.[3]

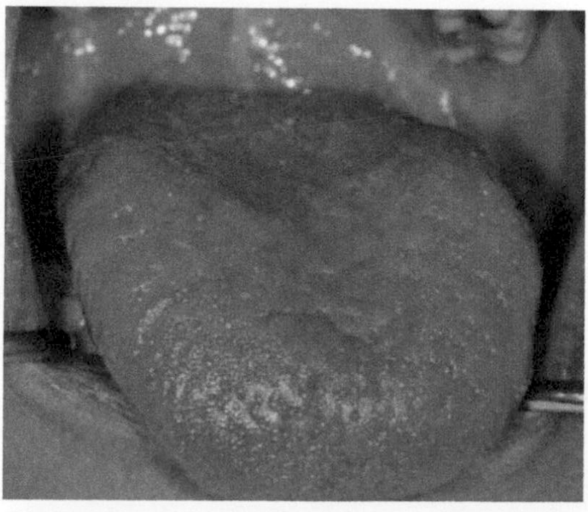

Fig. 2. Depapillated and dry dorsum of the tongue in a patient with hyposalivation after radioactive iodine therapy for managing hyperthyroidism. (*Courtesy of* Sahar Mirfarsi, DDS.)

CLINICS CARE POINTS

- Obtain medical records in patients with hyperthyroidism.
- Monitor vital signs before and during dental procedures to avoid complication.
- Most patients undergoing minor dental procedures with local anesthetic will not require corticosteroid supplementation.
- OHCPs should be aware of the adverse effects of radioactive iodine on the salivary glands, such as hyposalivation.
- Be cautious using epinephrine in local anesthetic or retraction cords in patients with hyperthyroidism.
- Take extreme caution administering epinephrine in local anesthetic to patients taking nonselective β-blockers.

DISCLOSURE

The authors have nothing to disclose.

REFERENCES

1. Glick M, Greenberg MS, Lockhart PB, et al. In: Burket's oral medicine. 13th edition. Hoboken, NJ: Wiley-Blackwell; 2021. p. 817–902. https://doi.org/10.1002/9781119597797.ch22.
2. Farag AM. Head and neck manifestations of endocrine disorders. Atlas Oral Maxillofac Surg Clin North Am 2017;25(2). https://doi.org/10.1016/j.cxom.2017.04.011.
3. Little JW. Thyroid disorders. Part I: hyperthyroidism. Oral Surg Oral Med Oral Pathol Oral Radiol Endod 2006;101(3):276–84. https://doi.org/10.1016/j.tripleo.2005.05.069.
4. Chandna S, Bathla M. Oral manifestations of thyroid disorders and its management. Indian J Endocrinol Metab 2011;15(6):113.
5. Hersh E v, Moore PA. Three serious drug interactions that every dentist should know about. Compend Contin Educ Dent 2015;36(6):408–13 [quiz: 414], 416.

Mandibular Jaw Lesion Excisional Biopsy on a Patient with Hyperparathyroidism (Primary)

Sahar Mirfarsi, DDS[a,*], Dalia Seleem, DDS, PhD[a],
Airani Sathananthan, MD[b]

KEYWORDS

- Primary hyperparathyroidism • Endocrine disease • Oral health care providers
- Excisional oral biopsy • Jaw lesion

KEY POINTS

- Most of the primary hyperparathyroidism is due to adenomas in the parathyroid glands.
- Hypercalcemia is more common in primary hyperparathyroidism.
- Hyperparathyroidism may be asymptomatic and detected incidentally as part of a routine serological evaluation.
- Oral health care providers should recognize distinct changes in the jawbone associated with primary and secondary hyperparathyroidism.

MEDICAL SCENARIO

A 62-year-old Hispanic woman is referred to a local oral and maxillofacial surgery office by her general dentist to evaluate a right anterior jaw lesion. The patient is asymptomatic, and her panoramic radiograph (**Fig. 1**) reveals a unilocular periapical radiolucency in the right mandibular incisor (tooth #25) area (**Fig. 2**). In addition, the dental pulp vitality tests on teeth #24, 25 and 26 confirm that all teeth are vital. Her family history is noncontributory.

Vital Signs

Blood pressure: 155/94 mm Hg.
Pulse: 92 beats per minute.

[a] Western University of Health Sciences, College of Dental Medicine, 309 East Second Street, Pomona, CA 91766-1854, USA; [b] Western University of Health Sciences, College of Osteopathic Medicine of the Pacific, Department of Internal Medicine, 309 East Second Street, Pomona, CA 91766-1854, USA
* Corresponding author. Western University of Health Sciences, College of Dental Medicine, 309 East Second Street, Pomona, CA 91766-1854.
E-mail address: Sahar.Mirfarsi@westernu.edu

Dent Clin N Am 67 (2023) 597–600
https://doi.org/10.1016/j.cden.2023.05.009
0011-8532/23/
dental.theclinics.com

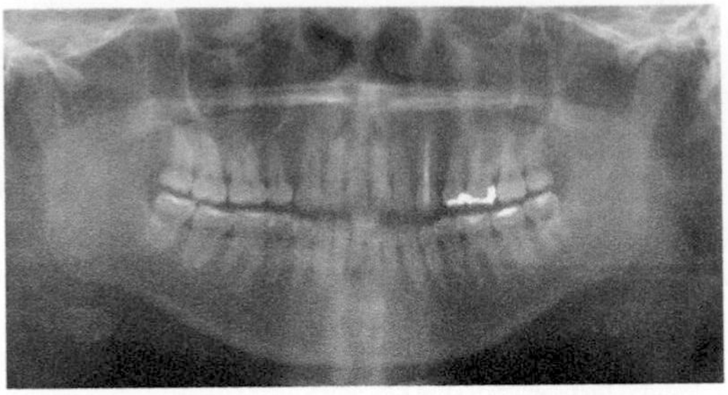

Fig. 1. Unilocular radiolucency in the anterior right mandibular, around the apex of tooth #25. (*Courtesy of* Sahar Mirfarsi, DDS.)

She recently established care with a primary care physician after a recent episode of nephrolithiasis.

Recent Laboratory Values

Serum calcium: 10.8 mg/dL (normal range: 8.6–10.3 mg/dL).

Serum phosphate: 1.8 mg/dL (normal range: 3.4–4.5 mg/dL).

Serum PTH: 142 pg/mL (normal range: 14–72 pg/mL).

Estimated glomerular filtration rate: 93 mL/min/1.73 m^2 (normal range for adults: >90 mL/min/1.73 m^2).

Her physician ordered a parathyroid sestamibi scan, revealing a possible right lower lobe parathyroid adenoma. On today's examination, she is asymptomatic, and there are no other abnormalities in her review of systems.

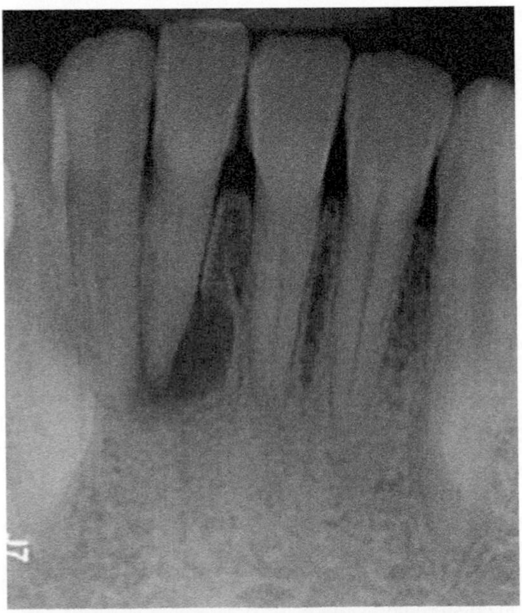

Fig. 2. Well-circumcised periapical radiolucency extending to the lateral mesial root of the mandibular anterior right incisor, tooth #25.

DENTAL MANAGEMENT DECISION AND JUSTIFICATION

Primary hyperparathyroidism is referred to as chronic overproduction of PTH by the parathyroid glands, which results in increased serum calcium or hypercalcemia.[1] Adenomas in the parathyroid glands are responsible for 80% of primary hyperparathyroidism cases.[2] Chronic kidney disease (CKD) can cause secondary hyperparathyroidism with an estimated prevalence of 8 to 6% globally.[3] Unlike primary hyperparathyroidism, hypocalcemia is seen in secondary hyperparathyroidism.[1] Primary hyperparathyroidism is more common in postmenopausal women.[4]

Patients with primary hyperparathyroidism may be asymptomatic. Initial findings can be incidental, with serum testing showing excess PTH production, elevated calcium serum level, low serum phosphate, and elevated alkaline phosphatase.[4] Skeletal manifestations from hyperparathyroidism include osteopenia or osteoporosis, which may be identified on dual-energy x-ray absorptiometry scanning.[5] Symptomatic manifestations of primary hyperparathyroidism can include nephrolithiasis and fractures.[4] Craniofacial bones, such as the jaw, can also be affected.[3] Maxilla and mandibular bones can present with diminished cortical bone, especially in the inferior border of the mandible. In severe cases, during heavy mechanical pressure from dental procedures, mandibular jawbone fractures[3] may result as a potential complication.[5]

Primary hyperparathyroidism can manifest as jawbone abnormalities[3] such as narrowing of dental pulp chambers, loss of lamina dura around the root of teeth, alterations in trabecular bone density often characterized as a "ground glass appearance," osteodystrophy, and leontiasis osteitis.[4] Brown tumors present as unilocular or multilocular maxillary and mandibular osseous radiolucency.[4] Osteitis fibrosa cystica is a condition that develops from the central degeneration and fibrosis of long-standing brown tumors.[3] Brown tumors are more common in the mandible than the maxilla and are pathognomonic of secondary hyperparathyroidism caused by CKD.[4] In general, brown tumors do not present with pain unless the bony changes cause bone expansion.[4] Therefore, ill-fitting and/or nonfitting removable dental prostheses in older patients or patients with CKD may prompt OHCP to screen for hyperparathyroidism.

For further histological analysis, an excisional biopsy of brown tumors is indicated in symptomatic patients and may reveal central giant cell granulomas (CGCG) in the jaw.[1] CGCG is a benign tumorlike lesion characterized by a proliferation of exceedingly vascular granulation tissue, which serves as a background for numerous multinucleated osteoclast-type giant cells.[1]

An interdisciplinary approach is necessary to manage patients with hyperparathyroidism. Addressing the underlying cause of hyperparathyroidism, related-systemic complications, and surgical excision of bony lesions may be required.[4] Patients with hyperparathyroidism may have poor bone healing; therefore, consulting physicians before dental surgical procedures may be beneficial to avoid dentoalveolar infections.[4] Bony alterations can elevate the risk of jaw fracture, cause orofacial disfiguration, and compromise normal functions such as mastication, compression, phonation, and the patient's quality of life.[1]

Surgical parathyroidectomy is the definitive medical treatment of patients with symptomatic primary hyperparathyroidism.[5] In addition to surgery, medical management may include antiresorptive medications such as bisphosphonates.[5] In such cases, the OHCP should be vigilant regarding the risk of developing medication-related osteonecrosis in the jaw.[5]

CLINICS CARE POINTS

- Take caution with dental surgical procedures on patients taking antiresorptive medications such as bisphosphonates.
- Poor bone healing is a risk factor in patients with hyperparathyroidism.
- Ill-fitting removable dental prostheses in older patients should prompt OHCPs to screen for hyperparathyroidism.
- Jaw fractures can happen due to bone alterations.

DISCLOSURE

The authors have nothing to disclose.

REFERENCES

1. Farag AM. Head and neck manifestations of endocrine disorders. Atlas Oral Maxillofac Surg Clin North Am 2017;25(2). https://doi.org/10.1016/j.cxom.2017.04.011.
2. Guimarães LM, Valeriano AT, Rebelo Pontes HA, et al. Manifestations of hyperparathyroidism in the jaws: Concepts, mechanisms, and clinical aspects. Oral Surg Oral Med Oral Pathol Oral Radiol 2022;133(5). https://doi.org/10.1016/j.oooo.2021.08.020.
3. Guimarães LM, Valeriano AT, Rebelo Pontes HA, et al. Manifestations of hyperparathyroidism in the jaws: concepts, mechanisms, and clinical aspects. Oral Surg Oral Med Oral Pathol Oral Radiol 2022;133(5):547–55.
4. Thoppay JR, Sollecito TP, De Rossi SS. Oral Signs of Endocrine and Metabolic Diseases. In: Fazel N, editor. Oral Signs of Systemic Disease. Cham: Springer; 2019. https://doi.org/10.1007/978-3-030-10863-2_4.
5. Glick M, Greenberg MS, Lockhart PB, et al. In: *Burket's oral medicine*. 13th edition. Hoboken, NJ: Wiley-Blackwell; 2021. p. 817–902. https://doi.org/10.1002/9781119597797.ch22.

A Patient with Hypothyroidism in Need of Periodontal Connective Tissue Graft Surgery

Sara N. Aldosary, BDS[a], Payam Mirfendereski, DDS[a],
Mel Mupparapu, DMD, MDS, Dipl ABOMR[b,*]

KEYWORDS

• Hypothyroidism • Myxedema • Myxedematous coma • Periodontitis

KEY POINTS

- Hypothyroidism is associated with various cardiovascular complications including hypercholesterolemia, arteriosclerosis, atrial fibrillation.
- Hypothyroidism is associated with a poor periodontal health due to decreased bone turnover, delayed tissue healing, and increased risk of infection.
- Hypothyroidism can present in the oral cavity as macroglossia, dysgeusia, delayed eruption of teeth, and altered tooth morphology.
- Myxedematous coma is a medical emergency that can arise in longstanding untreated hypothyroidism that requires rapid hospitalization and medical support.

MEDICAL SCENARIO

A 67-year-old female presents to the dental clinic with a complaint of anterior maxillary gingival recession with esthetic concerns. Her medical history is significant for hypothyroidism, hypercholesterolemia, and atrial fibrillation. She is currently taking levothyroxine 125 mcg daily, atorvastatin 40 mg daily, and apixaban 5 mg twice a day. Her family and social history are non-contributory. Radiographic examination reveals mild to moderate generalized marginal periodontitis. Extraoral examination revealed no lymphadenopathy or neurologic deficits. Intraoral examination revealed generalized mild calculus buildup and marginal gingival erythema as well as significant gingival recession in the labial gingiva of the maxillary central incisors. After comprehensive evaluation and treatment planning, the patient elected to proceed

[a] Department of Oral Medicine, University of Pennsylvania School of Dental Medicine, 240 South 40th Street, Philadelphia, PA 19104, USA; [b] Penn Dental Medicine
* Corresponding author.
E-mail address: mmd@upenn.edu

Dent Clin N Am 67 (2023) 601–603
https://doi.org/10.1016/j.cden.2023.05.017
dental.theclinics.com

with a multi-phased treatment plan encompassing periodontal connective tissue graft surgery to address her chief complaint of anterior maxillary gingival recession.

Dental Management Decision and Justification

The patient was referred to the periodontics clinic for the evaluation of the gingival recession and potential surgical intervention. Upon further clinical and radiographic evaluation, periodontal connective tissue graft surgery has been planned. Given that the patient has hypothyroidism, several factors must be taken into consideration during the patient's management.

Hypothyroidism is a condition for which the thyroid hormone is produced insufficiently from the thyroid gland that is not able to meet peripheral tissue requirements.[1] Primary hypothyroidism is the most common and accounts for about 99% of the cases which results from failure of the thyroid gland due to a certain disease or a condition, with a prevalence of 0.3%–3.7% in the United States.[1] The most common etiologies of primary hypothyroidism include chronic lymphocytic thyroiditis (Hashimoto's thyroiditis), radioiodine thyroid ablation, thyroidectomy, and high-dose head and neck radiation therapy.[1] The standard treatment for hypothyroidism is synthetic thyroid hormone replacement with levothyroxine.

In adults, longstanding hypothyroidism presents as myxedema, which is marked by slower metabolism, increased weight, edema, depressed mood, decreased pulse and respiratory rate, dry skin, and brittle hair. Hypothyroidism is associated with anemia, hypercholesterolemia, and arteriosclerosis and can lead to cardiac complications including sinus bradycardia, atrial fibrillation, and heart failure.[2]

Hypothyroidism can have varying oral manifestations in children and adults. Common oral findings that can be seen in patients with hypothyroidism include macroglossia, dysgeusia, delayed the eruption of teeth, poor periodontal health, altered tooth morphology, and delayed wound healing.[3] The increased incidence of periodontal disease in patients with hypothyroid has been associated with decreased bone turnover rate.[4] Hypothyroidism has also been associated with muscle weakness and myopathy, and Hashimoto's thyroiditis in particular has been associated with a higher prevalence of TMJ disorders.[5]

There are factors that should be considered during the dental management of patients with hypothyroidism[3].

1. It is important to obtain the patient's recent laboratory values including thyroid function tests and complete blood count to establish the level of control of the disease. A consultation with the patient's endocrinologist can be made in case of uncertainty.
2. Delayed healing due to decreased metabolic activity in fibroblasts might lead to an increased risk of infection due to longer exposure of unhealed tissue to pathogenic organisms.
3. Sedatives, narcotics, and other medications that induce central nervous system depression should be used with caution in patients with severe hypothyroidism given the possibility of respiratory depression.[2]
4. The dental provider should be aware of the possibility of myxedematous coma, a medical emergency that may occur in patients with untreated hypothyroidism. Signs and symptoms of myxedematous coma include altered mental status, weakness, lethargy, hypothermia, hypoxia, and hypoventilation.[6] After the diagnosis of myxedematous coma, the patient should be immediately transferred to the hospital setting for thyroid hormone administration and appropriate pulmonary and cardiovascular support.

5. In patients with hypothyroidism who do not have cardiovascular complications, the use of epinephrine-containing local anesthetic is not a concern, but caution should be employed in patients with greater cardiac involvement. Similarly, additional hemostatic measures are only considered in hyperthyroidism when concomitant cardiovascular complications necessitate anticoagulative therapy. For the patient above who has atrial fibrillation managed by apixaban, epinephrine should be used with caution and surgical trauma and procedural stress should be minimized as far as possible. Conservative hemostatic measures such as topical coagulating agents are typically sufficient.

CLINICS CARE POINTS

- Hypothyroidism can be often undiagnosed or underdiagnosed and it is essential to obtain history, physical evaluation and laboratory tests including thyroid function tests and complete blood count to establish the level of thyroid function if suspected before dental treatment.
- Delayed healing and risk of infection are possible complications if dental surgery is performed in patients with hypothyroidism.
- Respiratory depression is a possible complication in patients with hypothyroidism if sedatives, narcotics and similar agents are used that induce central nervous system depression.
- Caution needed when administering local anesthesia to hypothyroid patients who may have cardiovascular complications.

CONFLICT OF INTEREST

All authors declare that they have no commercial or financial conflict of interest related to the material in this article and have received no funding for the preparation of this article.

REFERENCES

1. McDermott Michael T. Hypothyroidism. Annals of internal medicine 2020;173(1): ITC1–16.
2. Pinto A, Glick M. Management of patients with thyroid disease: oral health considerations. J Am Dent Assoc 2002;133(7):849–58.
3. Chandna S, Bathla M. Oral manifestations of thyroid disorders and its management. Indian J Endocrinol Metab 2011;15(Suppl 2):S113–6.
4. Aldulaijan HA, Cohen RE, Stellrecht EM, et al. Relationship between hypothyroidism and periodontitis: A scoping review. Clin Exp Dent Res 2020;6(1):147–57.
5. Grozdinska A, Hofmann E, Schmid M, et al. Prevalence of temporomandibular disorders in patients with Hashimoto thyroiditis. Prävalenz von kraniomandibulären Dysfunktionen bei Patienten mit Hashimoto-Thyreoiditis. J Orofac Orthop 2018; 79(4):277–88.
6. Elshimy G, Chippa V, Correa R. Myxedema. [Updated 2023 Apr 16]. In: StatPearls [Internet]. Treasure Island (FL): StatPearls Publishing; 2023. p. 1–20. Available at: https://www.ncbi.nlm.nih.gov/books/NBK545193/.

The Patient Faints in the Waiting Area with a Suspected Hypoglycemic Event

Milda Chmieliauskaite, DMD, MPH[a,*],
Marie D. Grosh, DNP, APRN-CNP, LNHA[b], Ali Syed, BDS, MHA, MS[c],
Andres Pinto, DMD, MPH, MSCE, MBA[c]

KEYWORDS

• Diabetes • Hypoglycemia • Emergency • Dentist office

KEY POINTS

- Hypoglycemia is defined as a blood glucose level less than 70 mg/dL.
- Sulfonylurea drugs have a high risk of causing hypoglycemia in all users.
- Patients prescribed high-risk medications should be educated on safe use, and clinicians should assess the risk of hypoglycemia for each individual patient.

MEDICAL SCENARIO

An 80-year-old female presents to the clinic for an afternoon appointment for a denture adjustment with a past medical history of hypertension, hyperlipidemia, and type two diabetes mellitus. A senior transportation service dropped off the patient just after the lunch hour and the clinician is behind schedule. The patient proceeds to wait in the clinic's waiting area. Front-desk staff notices the patient is irritable and goes to check if the dentist is ready, they return and find the patient has slipped off the chair. The patient's eyes are open, but she seems confused, is slurring her words and slow to respond. A spot glucose is 54 mg/dL. Orange juice is administered, and other vitals are taken which are all within normal limits. The patient's glucose is rechecked 15 minutes later and is 115. Upon post-event interview with the patient she reveals that her type two diabetes is controlled with metformin 1000 mg twice daily and glipizide 5 mg twice daily. Today, the patient took all of her medication as

[a] UW Department of Oral Medicine School of Dentistry, Box 356370, 1959 NE Pacific Street, Seattle, WA 98195-6370, USA; [b] Frances Payne Bolton School of Nursing at Case Western Reserve University, Health Education Campus, 10900 Euclid Avenue, Cleveland, OH 44106-7343, USA; [c] School of Dental Medicine at Case Western Reserve University, Health Education Campus, 10900 Euclid Avenue, Cleveland, OH 44106-7343, USA
* Corresponding author. UW Department of Oral Medicine School of Dentistry, Box 356370, 1959 NE Pacific Street, Seattle, WA 98195-6370
E-mail address: mildac@uw.edu

Dent Clin N Am 67 (2023) 605–607
https://doi.org/10.1016/j.cden.2023.05.010
dental.theclinics.com
0011-8532/23/

prescribed. Her diet history for the day included a breakfast of cereal at 9 AM, and she has not eaten lunch yet because she is meeting a friend for lunch after her appointment. She took her Glipizide at noon today.

Dental Management Decision and Justification

Clinicians must be able to assess the risk of hypoglycemia for a patient with diabetes. The American Diabetes Association defines hypoglycemia in patients with diabetes as a blood glucose level less than 70 mg/dL.[1] In this scenario, the patient experienced a severe hypoglcemic event requiring active administration of a glycemic substance. In addition to reviewing the patient's demographics, medical history, and medications, appropriate follow-up questions will identify risk factors for hypoglycemia including: older age, recent history of hypoglycemia, food insecurity, insulin or sulfonylurea use, recent intensification or change of drug therapy, longer duration of diabetes, chronic kidney disease, alcoholism, hypoglycemia unawareness and meal skipping.[1] At each visit patients should be asked about meals and when or if they took their diabetes medications.[2]

Glipizide, a sulfonylurea, works by inducing spontaneous insulin release from pancreatic beta cells regardless of any endogenous feedback from blood glucose levels or food intake. Therefore, sulfonylureas are a class of medication that are at very high risk for causing hypoglycemia in all users. The American Geriatrics Society (AGS) publishes a Beers Criteria list of medications that should be avoided in older adults because of their high risk of harm in this population.[3] The list includes a strong recommendation to avoid long-acting sulfonylureas.[4] This is due to older adults' propensity to have other comorbidities, have catastrophic sequelae from a fall caused by hypoglycemia, and sluggish hepatic glucose response to hypoglycemia. Tools have been created to use electronic health record data to predict the 3-month risk of severe hypoglycaemia for individual patients.[4]

Clinicians caring for patients with diabetes should know how to recognize the signs and symptoms of a hypoglycemic reaction (**Box 1**). A glucometer is needed to assess for hyper- and hypoglycemia, and exogenous glucose to respond to a hypoglycemic episode. Patients who can swallow can be given 15 g of sugar.[1] The quickest way to

Box 1
Commonly associated signs and symptoms of low blood sugar

Early hypoglycemia	• Rapid heart rate • Light-headedness • Weakness • Sweating, especially palms of hands • Numbness and tingling in extremities • Dry mouth
Worsening hypoglycemia	Above symptoms and one of the following: • Disorientation/confusion • Agitation/anxiety • Trouble with word finding/slurred speech
Late/severe hypoglycemia	Above symptoms and one of the following: • Difficulty responding/unresponsiveness • Cold sweaty skin • Worsening tachycardia with irregular rhythm • Seizure activity

absorb sugar is through liquid forms (juice), which should be used first line. Solid forms such as cake frosting, crackers, or cookies can also used, but are slower to absorb. If a patient becomes unconscious, it is contraindicated to place anything that needs to be swallowed in the mouth due to a choking risk.[2] Glucose tabs or gels placed on the buccal mucosa are an option. Patients prescribed high-risk medications should be educated on safe use, and a clinician who witnesses a hypoglycemic episode should report it directly to the prescriber.

CLINICS CARE POINTS

- Long-acting sulfonylureas are listed in the American Geriatrics Society (AGS) published Beers Criteria list of medications that should be avoided in older adults due to their high risk of hypoglycemia.
- Conscious patients experiencing a hypoglycemic event should be given liquid forms of sugar (15g) first line.
- Patients that should not be given anything by mouth (i.e unconscious, choking risk) can be given glucose tabs or gels on the buccal mucosa.

REFERENCES

1. Cryer PE. Hypoglycemia in adults with diabetes mellitus. In: Hirsch IB, Rubinow K, editors. UpToDate. 2022. Available at: https://www.uptodate.com/contents/hypoglycemia-in-adults-with-diabetes-mellitus#!. Accessed June 21, 2023.
2. Little JW, Falace DA, Miller CS, et al. Chapter 14 - diabetes mellitus. In: Little JW, Falace DA, Miller CS, et al, editors. Little and falace's dental management of the medically compromised patient. Eighth Edition. St. Louis: Mosby; 2013. p. 219–39.
3. American Geriatrics Society. Updated AGS beers criteria® for potentially inappropriate medication use in older adults. J Am Geriatr Soc 2019;67:674–94.
4. Karter AJ, Warton EM, Lipska KJ, et al. Development and validation of a tool to identify patients with type 2 diabetes at high risk of hypoglycemia-related emergency department or hospital use. JAMA Intern Med 2017;177:1461–70.

An Elderly Patient with Undiagnosed Type 2 Diabetes Mellitus Presenting for an Emergency Extraction

Milda Chmieliauskaite, DMD, MPH[a,b,*],
Marie D. Grosh, DNP, APRN-CNP, LNHA[c], Ali Syed, BDS, MHA, MS[d],
Andres Pinto, DMD, MPH, MSCE, MBA[d]

KEYWORDS:

- Dental extraction • Diabetes • Screening • Dentist

KEY POINTS

- Diabetes is a risk factor for periodontal disease.
- Screening for diabetes should begin at age 35 years and can be earlier in the presence of comorbid risk factors.
- Screening can be easily performed by either a point-of-care fingerstick hemoglobin A1c or point glucose with a blood sugar meter.

MEDICAL SCENARIO

A 67-year-old Asian American male patient had a premolar extracted and was sent home without complications, only to return to the office 2 weeks later for follow-up of delayed healing at the extraction site. Previously, he was referred by the emergency department (ED) to the dentist for extraction of tooth #4, which was tender to percussion and palpation, had class III mobility, and moderate to severe generalized bone-loss was noted in the upper right quadrant. The patient does not have a dental or medical provider and no health insurance. He reports no medical history and no maintenance medications, he finished amoxicillin prescribed by the ED 3 weeks ago. His family history is significant for hypertension, cholesterolemia, myocardial infarction,

[a] University of Washington School of Dentistry, Box 356370, 1959 Northeast Pacific Street HSB-317C, Seattle, WA 98195-6370, USA; [b] Case Western Reserve University in Cleveland, OH, USA; [c] Frances Payne Bolton School of Nursing at Case Western Reserve University, Health Education Campus, 10900 Euclid Avenue, Cleveland, OH 44106-7343, USA; [d] School of Dental Medicine at Case Western Reserve University, Health Education Campus, 10900 Euclid Avenue, Cleveland, OH 44106-7343, USA
* Corresponding author.
E-mail address: mildac@uw.edu

Dent Clin N Am 67 (2023) 609–611
https://doi.org/10.1016/j.cden.2023.05.011
dental.theclinics.com

stroke, and diabetes. On examination he was 5′ 6″ and 150 lbs (body mass index [BMI] 24), and blood pressure was 145/90 mm Hg with a normal pulse, respiratory rate, and temperature. He reports no other symptoms on a review of systems.

DENTAL MANAGEMENT DECISION AND JUSTIFICATION

An estimated 8.5 million individuals in the United States have undiagnosed diabetes, and 75% of people with diabetes receive a late diagnosis after experiencing a comorbidity or complication.[1] However, an estimated 8% of the US population (~26 million people) will visit their dentist but not their medical provider in the same year, thus presenting an opportunity for diabetes screening in the dental office.[1] The American Diabetes Association (ADA) recommends screening to begin at age 35 years and can be intensified in the presence of comorbid risk factors: BMI greater than or equal to 25 kg/m^2 or greater than or equal to 23 kg/m^2 in Asian American persons and one or more additional risk factor (**Box 1**).[2] The ADA has also created a diabetes risk test for patients and providers.[2] Patients do not experience symptoms of type 2 diabetes until very late stages, making screening even more critical. Screening can be easily performed by either a point-of-care fingerstick hemoglobin A1c (HbA1c) or point glucose with a blood sugar meter. Blood sugar meters can be obtained at any over-the-counter pharmacy, are relatively inexpensive, and have no special storage requirements. A point glucose should always be interpreted in the context of the patient's fasting/postprandial state (see **Box 1**). Point-of-care HBa1C test kits can be obtained through medical supply vendors and have refrigeration requirements for storage and short shelf lives.

The American Dental Association recognizes that dentists have a role in screening for diabetes and that in-office monitoring of blood sugar control may aid in dental treatment planning with corresponding dental billing codes (ie, D0411, D0412) for such procedures.[3] Dental clinicians must feel comfortable communicating the meaning of the test results to patients if detected and quickly referring patients to a primary care provider for confirmatory testing with a second test without delay.[2] Also, explicitly linking signs and symptoms, such as this patient's periodontal disease, poor healing, and infections, to the test results can make your communications more compelling.

Box 1
Risk factors, laboratory values, and recommended action steps for diabetes screening

Test	Prediabetes	Diabetes	Recommended Action
A1C	5.7%–6.4% (39–47 mmol/mol)	≥6.5% (48 mmol/mol)	Refer to PCP
Fasting[a] plasma glucose	100–125 mg/dL (5.6–6.9 mmol/L)	≥126 mg/dL (7.0 mmol/L)	<400 mg/dL refer to PCP ≥400 mg/dL or signs/ symptoms[b] of DKA transfer to ED
Random plasma glucose in a patient with symptoms of hyperglycemia	—	≥200 mg/dL (11.1 mmol/L)	<400 mg/dL refer to PCP ≥400 mg/dL or signs/ symptoms[a] of DKA transfer to ED

Abbreviations: DKA, diabetic ketoacidosis; ED, emergency department; PCP, primary care provider. [a]Fasting: no calorie intake for greater than 8 h. [b]Signs and symptoms of DKA: fast deep breathing, dry skin/mouth, flushed face, fruity-smelling breath, headache, muscle stiffness or aches, fatigue, nausea/vomiting, stomach pain.

Patients with a plasma glucose greater than 400 mg/dL or signs/symptoms of diabetic ketoacidosis (see **Box 1**) should be sent to the ED for management.

In this scenario, this patient presented with multiple risk factors for diabetes as well as periodontal disease. His undiagnosed diabetes is a significant contributor to the severity of his periodontal disease and will continue to cause further systemic and oral health complications if left untreated.

RISK FACTORS FOR DIABETES

- First-degree relative with diabetes
- High-risk race/ethnicity (eg, African American, Latino, Native American, Asian American, Pacific Islander)
- History of cardiovascular disease
- Hypertension (≥140/90 mm Hg or on therapy for hypertension)
- High-density lipoprotein cholesterol level less than 35 mg/dL (0.90 mmol/L) and/or a triglyceride level greater than 250 mg/dL (2.82 mmol/L)
- Women with polycystic ovary syndrome
- Physical inactivity
- Other clinical conditions associated with insulin resistance (eg, severe obesity, acanthosis nigricans)

CLINICS CARE POINTS

- The American Diabetes Association (ADA) recommends screening for diabetes to begin at age 35 years.
- Individuals with plasma glucose >400 mg/dL or signs/symptoms of diabetic ketoacidosis should be sent to the emergency department for management.

REFERENCES

1. Estrich CG, Araujo MWB, Lipman RD. Prediabetes and Diabetes Screening in Dental Care Settings: NHANES 2013 to 2016. JDR Clin Trans Res 2019;4(1):76–85.
2. American Dental Association. Standards of Medical Care in Diabetes—2022 Abridged for Primary Care Providers. Clin Diabetes 2022;40(1):10–38.
3. D0411 and D0412 – ADA Quick Guide to In-Office Monitoring and Documenting Patient Blood Glucose and HbA1C Level. Available at: https://www.mouthhealthy.org/~/media/ADA/Publications/Files/CDT_D0411_D0412_Guide_v1_2019Jan02.pdf?la=en. Accessed on 09/09/2022.

A Diabetic Patient with a Recent History of Flap and Osseous Surgery Presents Back with Bleeding and Infection

Milda Chmieliauskaite, DMD, MPH[a,*],
Marie D. Grosh, DNP, APRN-CNP, LNHA[b], Ali Syed, BDS, MHA, MS[c],
Andres Pinto, DMD, MPH, MSCE, MBA[c]

KEYWORDS

- Bleeding • Diabetes • Renal disease • Infection • Postsurgical
- Periodontal disease • Periodontal treatment • Healing

KEY POINTS

- Poorly controlled diabetes and chronic kidney disease may predispose patients to increased postsurgical risks of infection and bleeding.
- Long-term glycemic control via an hemoglobin A1c should be assessed within 3 months of the planned periodontal surgical procedure.
- Chronic kidney disease is common in patients with diabetes and should be assessed preoperatively using estimated glomerular filtration rate.
- New Clinical Practice Guidelines for treatment of stage I to III periodontitis suggest a stepwise approach to periodontal therapy.

MEDICAL SCENARIO

A 55-year-old woman presents to the periodontist 7 days after open flap debridement and periodontal osseous surgery with bleeding and pain from the postoperative site in the bilateral maxillary quadrants. Her past dental history is significant for stage III periodontal disease. Medical history is significant for diabetes type II, renal disease, and hypertension. Medications include metformin and aspirin. Her vitals are: temperature 98.7 F, blood pressure 150/85 mm Hg, 101 pulse, normal respirations. Her BMI is 30.

[a] University of Washington, Department of Oral Medicine School of Dentistry, Box 356370, 1959 NE Pacific Street Seattle, WA 98195-6370, USA; [b] Frances Payne Bolton School of Nursing at Case Western Reserve University, Health Education Campus, 10900 Euclid Avenue, Cleveland, OH 44106-7343, USA; [c] School of Dental Medicine at Case Western Reserve University, Health Education Campus, 10900 Euclid Avenue, Cleveland, OH 44106-7343, USA
* Corresponding author.
E-mail address: mildac@uw.edu

Dent Clin N Am 67 (2023) 613–615
https://doi.org/10.1016/j.cden.2023.05.012
dental.theclinics.com

Her last hemoglobin A1c (HbA1c) measured 6 months ago was 7%. On physical examination she has purulent drainage from the gingiva on palpation with generalized erythema and light bleeding on touch.

DENTAL MANAGEMENT DECISION AND JUSTIFICATION

Evidence about the risk of postsurgical infection following periodontal procedures in patients with diabetes at varying levels of glycemic control is low.[1] However, there is evidence that patients with higher levels of preoperative blood glucose levels and poorly controlled diabetes are at risk for postoperative infection after surgery.[1,2] Postoperative complications of poor wound healing and increased risk of infection are thought to be related to decreased immune function and compromised circulation to tissues. In addition, individuals with diabetes are at increased risk for comorbidities (eg, cardiovascular, renal disease). This case demonstrates a patient whose medical conditions (ie, diabetes, renal disease) were not thoroughly assessed before surgery and contributed to her increased risk of postsurgical bleeding, infection, and subsequent poor healing.

There are no formal dental guidelines for preoperative assessment of patients with diabetes. In general, long-term levels of hyperglycemia should be assessed using the HbA1c that is within 3 months of the planned procedure.[1] The A1C gives an average of what a patient's blood sugar has been over the previous 3 months (**Table 1**). Chronic kidney disease (CKD) affects 1 in 3 adults with diabetes, which predisposes patients to impaired hemostasis and risk of infection.[1] The stage of CKD should be determined based on the estimated glomerular filtration rate (see **Table 1**).[1]

The American Diabetes Association does not recommend a threshold for HbA1c at which to withhold surgical procedures. HbA1c thresholds are typically published as relative contraindications to elective surgery with recommendation from the United Kingdom to achieve a preoperative HbA1c level of less than 8.5% when safe and possible.[2] However, risks and benefits of the procedure and individual patient factors must be considered. Often, it may not be possible or practical to delay procedures until optimal glycemic control is reached.

Table 1
HbA1c, estimated average glucose, and chronic kidney disease laboratory values

HbA1c	Estimated Average Glucose mg/dL
7	154
8	183
9	212
10	240
Stage of CKD	**eGFR**
1	≥ 90
2	60–89
3a	45–59
3b	30–44
4	15–29
5	<15

Abbreviations: CKD, chronic kidney disease; eGFR, estimated glomerular filtration rate.
Created using Refs.[1,4]

For example, in this case the dentist may consider performing the subgingival scaling and deferring the open flap osseous surgery to optimize glycemic control. The new Clinical Practice Guidelines for treatment of stage I to III periodontitis suggest a stepwise approach to therapy and recommend steps 1 (removing supragingival plaque and behavioral modifications to decrease risk factors for periodontitis) and 2 (subgingival instrumentation) for all 3 stages of periodontitis (I–III).[3] Only when areas are not responsive to steps 1 and 2 are more advanced surgical procedures of stage 3 considered.[3]

Although routine use of antibiotics in patients with diabetes presenting for dental surgery is not recommended, antibiotics may be considered for patients undergoing invasive procedures whose oral health is poor and fasting plasma glucose is greater than 200 mg/dL based on expert opinion.[1] Follow-up of patients and patient education on signs of infection may help to identify postoperative complications early. Surgical incision and drainage with sterile saline irrigation and removal of necrotic tissue and appropriate pain control is recommended. Treatment with systemic antibiotics can be considered when systemic signs of infection (elevated temperature) are present or in immunocompromised individuals.[1] Chlorhexidine gluconate 0.12% rinse twice a day may also be of benefit. Follow-up in 2 to 3 days by phone; if there is no improvement, consider changing the antibiotic class. In all cases reevaluate the patient in 1 week.

CLINICS CARE POINTS

- Routine use of antibiotics for dental surgery is not recommended.
- Antibiotics may be considered for invasive procedures when fasting plasma glucose is >200 mg/dL

REFERENCES

1. Little J, Miller C, Rhodus N. Diabetes In Little and Falace's Dental Management of the Medically Compromised Patient Ninth ed. St. Louis, Missouri: Eslevier, 2018, Available at: http://ezsecureaccess.balamand.edu.lb/login?url=https://www.clinicalkey.com/dura/browse/bookChapter/3-s2.0-C20150014228. Accessed September 20 2022.
2. Grant B, Chowdhury TA. New guidance on the perioperative management of diabetes. Clin Med (Lond) 2022;22(1):41–4.
3. Sanz M, Herrera D, Kebschull M, et al. Treatment of stage I-III periodontitis-The EFP S3 level clinical practice guideline. J Clin Periodontol 2020;47(Suppl 22):4–60.
4. A1C and eAG. Available at: https://diabetes.org/diabetes/a1c/a1c-and-eag. Accessed September 20, 2022.

Patient with Type I Diabetes Mellitus Develops Post-Operative Hyperglycemia After Osseous Surgery

Milda Chmieliauskaite, DMD, MPH[a,*],
Marie D. Grosh, DNP, APRN-CNP, LNHA[b], Ali Syed, BDS, MHA, MS[c],
Andres Pinto, DMD, MPH, MSCE, MBA[c]

KEYWORDS

- Diabetes • Hyperglycemia • Post-operative complications • Dental surgery
- Nutrition

KEY POINTS

- Hyperglycemia puts patients at risk for poor wound healing, infections, and, if severe, diabetic ketoacidosis (DKA).
- Extensive dental surgery may temporarily alter a patients' diet and communication with the patient and their endocrinologist may be necessary to ensure optimal glycemic control in the postoperative period.
- After outpatient surgery patients that take insulin should monitor glucose levels every 2 hours for several hours, while type two diabetics should monitor every 4 hours. A patient's physician should be notified if blood sugars are persistently >250 mg/dL.

MEDICAL SCENARIO

A 65-year-old female patient presents to her primary care provider for routine follow-up of type I diabetes mellitus. Two weeks prior she had outpatient osseous surgery including full mouth extraction with bimaxillary alveoplasty and tori removal under local anesthesia. After the surgery she reports trouble eating and modified her diet significantly towards liquid or very soft foods (ie, fruit smoothies, yogurt). She stopped taking her insulin the day of the dental procedure anticipating interference with normal

[a] University of Washington Department of Oral Medicine School of Dentistry, Box 356370, 1959 NE Pacific Street, Seattle, WA 98195-6370, USA; [b] Frances Payne Bolton School of Nursing at Case Western Reserve University, Health Education Campus, 10900 Euclid Avenue, Cleveland, OH 44106-7343, USA; [c] School of Dental Medicine at Case Western Reserve University, Health Education Campus, 10900 Euclid Avenue, Cleveland, OH 44106-7343, USA
* Corresponding author.
E-mail address: mildac@uw.edu

Dent Clin N Am 67 (2023) 617–619
https://doi.org/10.1016/j.cden.2023.05.013
dental.theclinics.com

eating post-operatively without consulting with her physician. Her medical history is significant for type I diabetes, hypertension, and glaucoma. Medications include insulin glargine 30 units once daily, humalog insulin preprandial boluses on a sliding scale, lisinopril 20 mg daily, and she has no allergies. On physical examination, her BMI is 24 and all vitals are stable. A point glucose is 295.

Dental Management Decision and Justification

Type one diabetes is characterized by the inability of the pancreas to produce insulin, therefore requiring exogenous insulin to meet both basal and prandial insulin needs. Withholding all forms of insulin, and replacing her otherwise diabetes conscious diet with fruit smoothies and yogurts (typically high in glucose), resulted in postoperative hyperglycemia. Hyperglycemic states are defined by a random glucose reading over 200 mg/dL. Hyperglycemia puts patients at risk for poor wound healing, infections, and, if severe, diabetic ketoacidosis (DKA).[1] Patients with blood sugars over 350 mg/DL may show signs and symptoms of DKA, including confusion, stupor, blurred vision, intense thirst, frequent urination, and breath with a fermented fruit odor from ketones, and dehydration. If DKA is suspected, transfer to an emergency room is appropriate so patients can have IV insulin to bring their blood sugar back into control and correct electrolyte imbalances.

Perioperative management of a patient with diabetes depends on the type of diabetes (I or II), level of glycemic control, extent of surgery, anesthesia, and co-morbid conditions.[2] Detailed recommendations for the perioperative management of patients have been published and **Fig. 1** summarizes factors that may lead towards hyper and hypoglycemia in the perioperative period.[2,3] However, it is also recommended that dental professionals collaborate with a patient's endocrinologist regarding perioperative management. Patients or dentists with insufficient training should not alter an individual's medication regimen without consulting the endocrinologist. Dental surgery may often result in patients not being able to resume their normal diet longer periods of time than may be common in other surgical procedures not affecting the head/neck. Communicating with patients and medical colleagues what the anticipated disruption in food intake may be and its length of time so that medications can be altered is often overlooked. Patients should be informed of guidelines for postoperative self-monitoring of blood glucose levels. Patients that take insulin should monitor glucose levels every 2 hours for several hours with algorithms provided by the endocrinologist for supplemental insulin administration.[4] In type two diabetes monitoring every 4 hours after outpatient surgery is sufficient.[4] Patients should contact their physician if blood glucose levels are persistently >250 mg/dL.[3] Many patients with type one diabetes have advanced technology insulin pump and continuous glucose monitoring (CGM) systems that

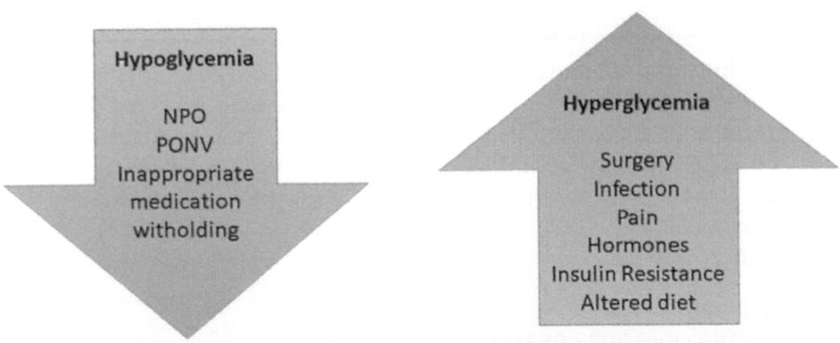

Fig. 1. Balancing perioperative glycemia. (*Adapted from* Ref.[4])

communicate wireless data to their endocrinologist. Advanced communication between providers prepares both parties to anticipate perioperative alterations in glucose control.

Regardless of food intake (ie, even in a fasting state), the human body requires basal insulin at all times to maintain normoglycemia by its long-acting (24–48 hours) suppression of hepatic glucose. A common reason for hospitalization for DKA in insulin-dependent patients involves individuals with low health literacy and/or knowledge deficits deciding to omit their basal insulin in transient states of interrupted oral intake such as perioperatively. Conversely, rapid-acting mealtime insulin (eg, lispro, aspart, glulisine) is given in pre-prandial boluses to digest food intake. Mealtime insulin is often recommended to be decreased or omitted during times of altered oral intake. Dental clinicians must be comfortable assessing insulin compliance by asking patients open-ended questions specifically regarding each kind of insulin (eg, basal v. bolus, short acting v long acting), when exactly the patient is taking each type (eg, morning/night-time v. mealtime), what their glucose readings have been, and what they have been eating/drinking.

CLINICS CARE POINTS

- The human body requires basal insulin regardless of food intake, while mealtime insulin may need to be altered during altered oral intake.
- Patients with blood sugars over 350 mg/DL and signs and symptoms of DKA should go to an emergency room to bring blood sugar back into control.

REFERENCES

1. Ata A, Lee J, Bestle SL, et al. Postoperative hyperglycemia and surgical site infection in general surgery patients. Arch Surg 2010;145(9):858–64.
2. Ead H. Glycemic control and surgery—optimizing outcomes for the patient with diabetes. J PeriAnesthesia Nurs 2009;24(6):384–95.
3. Bergman S. Perioperative management of the diabetic patient. Oral Surg Oral Med Oral Pathol Oral Radiol Endod 2007;103(6):731–7.
4. Marks JB. Perioperative management of diabetes. Am Fam Physician 2003;67(1): 93–100.

A Diabetic Patient with Acute Osteomyelitis Presenting with Jaw Pain and Submandibular Swelling

Mel Mupparapu, DMD, MDS, DiplABOMR[a,*],
Angela M. Barnes, RDH, PHDHP, MEd[b], Archana Mupparapu, BS[c],
Steven R. Singer, DDS[d]

KEYWORDS

• Osteomyelitis • Mandible • Jaw pain • Abscess • Inflammation
• Type 1 Diabetes Mellitus

KEY POINTS

- Management of type 1 diabetes mellitus.
- Identification of osteomyelitis.
- Management of osteomyelitis.
- Selection of antibiotic appropriate to the infection.
- Culture and sensitivity of the microbes.

MEDICAL SCENARIO

A 26-year-old female patient presents to Oral Medicine with jaw pain and right submandibular swelling. She has type 1 diabetes mellitus (T1D) managed by long-acting basal Insulin. Patient titers insulin at home every 2 or 3 days. No other medical comorbidities. Physical examination revealed a generalized swelling on the mandibular right side, teeth 28 to 30 sensitive to palpation.

DENTAL MANAGEMENT DECISION AND JUSTIFICATION

Patient presented with a fluctuant swelling on the right side of the jaw with pus discharge on palpation (**Fig. 1**) from intraoral sinuses in the vicinity of teeth 27, 28, 29, and 30 (mandibular right quadrant). All the teeth in the region were tender to

[a] University of Pennsylvania School of Dental Medicine; [b] Community College of Philadelphia; [c] Temple University School of Medicine; [d] Rutgers University School of Dental Medicine
* Corresponding author. Penn Dental Medicine, Dept of Oral Medicine, 240 S 40th Street, Philadelphia, PA 191104.
E-mail address: mmd@upenn.edu

Dent Clin N Am 67 (2023) 621–624
https://doi.org/10.1016/j.cden.2023.05.025
dental.theclinics.com

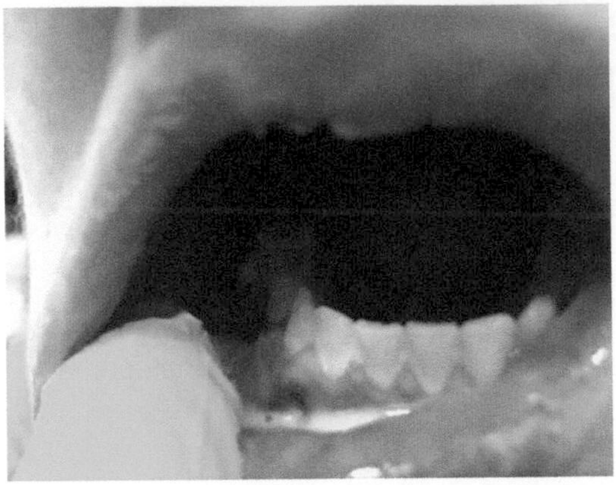

Fig. 1. Intraoral photograph of the patient showing pus discharge noted in the mouth from right mandibular infection.

palpation. Patient reported to Oral & Maxillofacial Surgery clinic where an incision and drainage was performed. A panoramic radiograph was obtained at this visit that demonstrated no significant bony changes. Patient was placed on clindamycin, 300 mg, every 6 hours for 5 days. Patient was referred to the Hospital of the University of Pennsylvania where a computed tomography (CT) of head and neck with contrast was obtained. The CT showed regions of low attenuation in the right submandibular and sublingual spaces abutting the lingual and buccal cortices of the right mandibular body. There were changes suggestive of acute inflammation and reported as abscess formation, with a differential diagnosis of infection secondary to a tooth decay. Pus collection in the region seen on the CT was documented. Right level 1B lymph node enlargement was also documented. A few days later, patient reported to the Emergency Room of Hospital of the University of Pennsylvania with significant pain and swelling of the right submandibular region. Both intraoral drainage and extraoral drainage were performed at the hospital, and clindamycin was continued for suspected submandibular/sublingual space infection. Patient was referred to the dental school for management of a suspected deep carious lesion and necrotic pulp of tooth 28. Clinical examination revealed unhealed sinuses actively draining pus at this visit. A cone-beam CT was ordered at this visit, which showed significant changes in the alveolar bone housing teeth 27, 28, and 29. There was generalized widening of the periodontal ligament space, mixed density areas of the alveolus, giving the bone a "moth-eaten" appearance. Both teeth 28 and 29 had deep carious lesions, but the lesion in tooth 29 seemed more widespread. Patient felt better after this appointment, as she completed the course of antibiotics and followed rigorous home care. The attending clinicians suspected tooth 30 to be the culprit and extracted that tooth. A head/neck CT with contrast taken a week later showed near complete resolution of the fluid collection along buccal and lingual cortices. The patient was dismissed with home care instructions. An MRI taken on the same day the CT was obtained showed evidence of right mandibular osteomyelitis, with decreased signal of the bone marrow in the region corresponding to 27, 28, and 29, suggesting decreased fluid content. Patient was reevaluated a week later and given a clean bill of health. A few days later, patient had a recurrence of the extraoral sinus tract and presented to the Hospital of the University of Pennsylvania for treatment (**Fig. 2**). A new panoramic radiograph taken at this visit revealed significant bone loss, loss of continuity of the mandibular inferior cortex, and what seemed to be a sequestrum and multiple

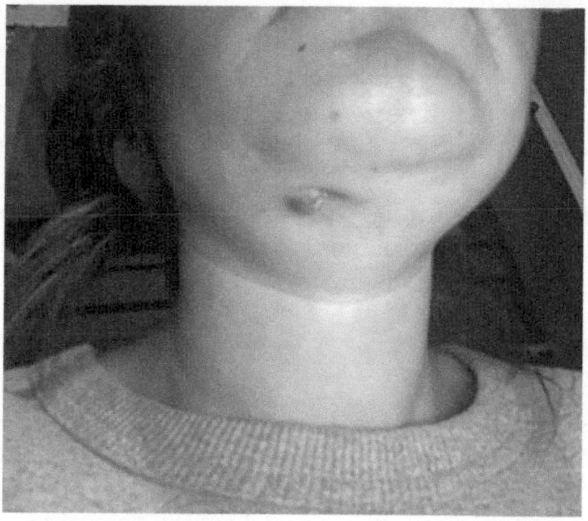

Fig. 2. Extraoral fistula noted midway through the treatment after a prior incision and drainage of the area.

ill-defined radiolucent foci apical to teeth 27, 28, and 29 (**Fig. 3**). At this time, the patient was admitted to the hospital for a culture and sensitivity of the discharge for appropriate antibiotic coverage, and deep curettage and clean-up of the necrotic bone in the region was also suggested.

Although the management of the patient seemed appropriate at given points of time, the patient continued to suffer without any resolution of the osteomyelitis. Further, tooth 29 could not be treated endodontically because there were acute flare-ups of the infection related to this tooth. Was tooth 30 a culprit at all? Why did Clindamycin not work? Would it be better if we had the culture and sensitivity done the first time, before prescribing antibiotics?

Ideal Management

Patients with T1D need to be managed carefully, especially if an odontogenic infection is present. They are more prone to periodontitis, as there is increased expression of inflammatory cytokines and RANKL, which promote bone resorption.[1,2] In addition, reduced anabolic activity in periodontal tissues impairs soft tissue and bone repair. It is vital to ensure the patient is managing blood glucose levels sufficiently with either long-acting insulin or insulin pumps. Insulin deficiency can lead to dangerous acute

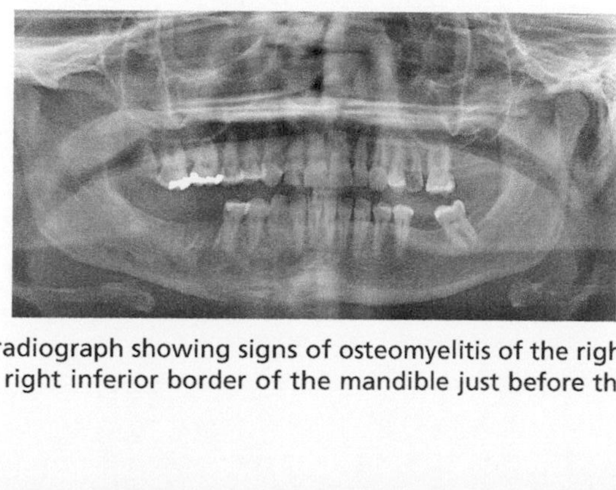

Fig. 3. Panoramic radiograph showing signs of osteomyelitis of the right mandible and the sequestrum of the right inferior border of the mandible just before the hospitalization of the patient.

conditions such as diabetic ketoacidosis and hyperosmolar hyperglycemic syndrome, both of which require urgent medical intervention. It is important, therefore, to closely monitor the patient's diabetic management and involve the patient's physician. When an osteomyelitis is suspected or known, the patient should be immediately hospitalized. Culture and sensitivity of the microbiota causing the infection must be identified and an appropriate antibiotic must be given.[3] Intravenous antibiotic administration is preferred. Oral antibiotics are not the choice of medication in cases complicated by underlying conditions such as diabetes, especially if an osteomyelitis is already set in.[3,4]

CLINICS CARE POINTS

- Dental patients with underlying Diabetes Mellitus need to be managed proactively as they are prone to periodontitis and odontogenic infections.
- When a jaw osteomyelitis is suspected in a dental patient, hospitalization is recommended for better monitoring, culture and sensitivity of the microbes involved and administration of parenteral antibiotics that would significantly improve overall health outcomes.

DISCLOSURE

None.

REFERENCES

1. Graves DT, Ding Z, Yang Y. The impact of diabetes on periodontal diseases. Periodontol 2000;82(1):214–24.
2. Genco RJ, Borgnakke WS. Diabetes as a potential risk for periodontitis: association studies. Periodontol 2000;83(1):40–5.
3. Moratin J, Freudlsperger C, Metzger K, et al. Development of osteomyelitis following dental abscesses-influence of therapy and comorbidities. Clin Oral Investig 2021;25(3):1395–401.
4. Andre CV, Khonsari RH, Ernenwein D, et al. Osteomyelitis of the jaws: A retrospective series of 40 patients. J Stomatol Oral Maxillofac Surg 2017;118(5):261–4.

A Patient with Juvenile Idiopathic Arthritis Presents for Dental Extraction

Roopali Kulkarni, DMD, MPH*, Sunday Akintoye, BDS, DDS, MS

KEYWORDS

• Juvenile idiopathic arthritis • Dental extraction • Temporomandibular joint

KEY POINTS

- Juvenile idiopathic arthritis (JIA) is the most common type of arthritis in children under the age of 16 years.
- Temporomandibular joint (TMJ) involvement is most commonly seen in the polyarticular subtype of JIA. Arthritis of the TMJ can result in pain and limitations in opening.
- Oral health and hygiene practices may be impacted by TMJ arthritis. As such, dental considerations must include education regarding the condition, routine dental care, review of oral hygiene practices, and nutrition counselling.
- Dental management includes considerations before treatment, during treatment, and after treatment. During treatment, frequent breaks may be needed, and appliances to support opening may be used to complete dental procedures effectively.
- When completing dental extractions in patients with JIA, bite blocks or mouth props can aid in reducing pressure on the jaw and aid in mouth opening.

MEDICAL SCENARIO

A 14-year-old female patient with seropositive polyarticular juvenile idiopathic arthritis (JIA) with bilateral temporomandibular joint (TMJ) involvement presents with her mother for extraction of nonrestorable #30.

DENTAL MANAGEMENT DECISION AND JUSTIFICATION

[Please add a paragraph or two about the different types of JIA noted among kids and the most common symptomatology when the condition is active, eg, … affecting eyes, bones, mouth and jaw, neck, skin, lungs. For audiences, this is a learning platform;

Department of Oral Medicine, University of Pennsylvania School of Dental Medicine, Philadelphia, PA, USA
* Corresponding author. 240 South 40th Street, Room 215, Philadelphia, PA 19104.
E-mail address: RoopaliK@upenn.edu

Dent Clin N Am 67 (2023) 625–628
https://doi.org/10.1016/j.cden.2023.06.001

hence, my suggestion would be to add the most common tests that the patient may be undergoing or having undergone, like ESR/CRP, ANA, RF, HLA B27, CBC, and imaging. Not all the tests are positive, or may be none are positive in some cases. Only RF is positive in some cases, as you mentioned in the scenario. This kind of puts the patient in a categorization that is a stable managed condition from the primary care now referred for an extraction. Alternately, you would see all the symptoms and not extract the tooth–also acceptable. JIA is the most common rheumatic disease of childhood, with unknown etiology. It is characterized by inflammation of the joints in individuals aged 16 years or younger. Chronic inflammation may limit daily activities and productivity. There are 7 subtypes of the condition, including oligoarticular, seropositive polyarticular, seronegative polyarticular, systemic-onset, enthesitis-related, juvenile psoriatic, and undifferentiated. The oligoarticular is the most common subtype, accounting for approximately 50% of cases that involve 4 or fewer joints. It tends to impact toddlers most often with uveitis and knee and ankle joint involvement. Polyarticular, which accounts for approximately 30% to 40% of cases, is defined as arthritis of 5 or more joints during the first 6 months of the disease. Rheumatoid factor may or may not be positive. Enthesitis-related is one of the most controversial topics in pediatric rheumatology, showing characteristics of both JIA and juvenile spondyloarthropathies. The psoriatic subtype is defined by arthritis with either a psoriatic rash or 2 of the following: dactylitis, nail pitting or onycholysis, or psoriasis in a first-degree relative.

Diagnosis of subtype is important for determining therapy options, follow-up strategies, and predicting prognosis. In addition to symptomatology, diagnostic tests may include rheumatoid factor, erythrocyte sedimentation rate, C-reactive protein, antinuclear antibody, HLA-B27 antigen testing, Lyme antibody test, complete blood count to assess for anemia, comprehensive metabolic panel, joint fluid analysis, and urinalysis. Imaging such as x-rays, ultrasound, or MRI may be indicated to assess joint damage or deformities.

A 14-year-old female patient presents with her mother to the dental clinic with a chief complaint of sharp pain on the lower right side for 5 days. The tooth in question is sensitive to both hot and cold. The pain is preventing the patient from sleeping. The patient has not taken any medications to help ease the pain. Past medical, social, and surgical history is noncontributory, excepting for seropositive polyarticular JIA, diagnosed four months prior to presentation. Medications included oral prednisone. Review of systems was significant for generalized joint pain in the knees, hips, and ankles.

The patient's mother reports irregular dental visits, poor oral hygiene, and frequent snacking. Due to bilateral jaw pain, the patient is unable to open wide. The patient's mother states that the primary goal is to eliminate the source of the pain.

An extraoral and intraoral head and neck examination and dental examination was completed. Extraoral examination did not reveal lymphadenopathy, and cranial nerves II-XII were grossly intact. Intraoral examination revealed #30 with a large carious lesion extending toward the pulp and fracture of the crown. Vitality testing of #30 revealed severe discomfort upon percussion, no significant pain upon palpation, and application of Endo-Ice resulted in lingering discomfort. A bitewing and periapical radiographs were obtained, which revealed grossly decayed #30.

Based on clinical and radiographic evaluation, #30 is deemed nonrestorable, with a plan for extraction under local anesthesia. Given the diagnosis of JIA and current prednisone use, blood pressure was monitored throughout the procedure, and a pediatric mouth prop was used during the procedure for ease of opening. The tooth was extracted in one unit without complications. The patient and the patient's mother were advised to follow-up in 2 weeks postextraction.

The patient and the patient's mother were counselled on the importance of general management of JIA, full evaluation of TMJs, and treatment as needed to aid in mouth opening. Both were educated on the importance of oral health, at-home hygiene regimen, and adequate nutritional intake. Additionally, they were counselled on the importance of resting the jaw and continuing follow-up to monitor opening.

HIGHLIGHTS AND ADDITIONAL CONSIDERATIONS

- Seropositive polyarticular JIA is one subtype, which typically affects 30% to 40% of those diagnosed with JIA. It is defined as arthritis of 5 or more joints during the first 6 months of the disease, and TMJ arthritis is present in the majority of the cases. As a result of the TMJ involvement, secondary microretrognathia is common.[1–3]
- Patients diagnosed with JIA may be on analgesics, corticosteroids, disease-modifying antirheumatic drugs, or biologic agents. It is important to understand the impact of pharmacologic management on the condition and additional dental considerations. In this case, corticosteroids may increase blood pressure and blood sugar, modify mood, and increase risk of infection.
- Limited mouth opening and pain upon opening wide can be a consequence of TMJ arthritis.[4,5]
- Long-term effects can include higher risk of dental caries, periodontal disease, and significant dysfunction of the jaw.[4]
- Treatment considerations for patients with JIA include frequent breaks during procedures, use of props or blocks to aid in mouth opening, and shorter dental visits.
- Long-term treatment considerations include multidisciplinary management of the JIA, more frequent periodontal maintenance appointments, and education on the importance of oral hygiene.

CLINICS CARE POINTS

- Shorter dental appointments and/or frequent breaks may be needed in patients with JIA.
- Mouth props/blocks may be useful for patients with JIA to aid in completing treatment while reducing pain.

DISCLOSURE

The authors have no disclosures.

REFERENCES

1. Okamoto N, Yokota S, Takei S, et al. Clinical practice guidance for juvenile idiopathic arthritis (JIA) 2018. Mod Rheumatol 2019;29(1):41–59.
2. Zaripova LN, Midgley A, Christmas SE. Juvenile idiopathic arthritis: from aetiopathogenesis to therapeutic approaches. Pediatr Rheumatol Online J 2021; 19(1):135.

3. Viscuso D, Storari M, Aprile M, et al. Temporomandibular disorders and juvenile idiopathic arthritis: Scoping review with a case report. Eur J Paediatr Dent 2020; 21(4):303–8.
4. Sahni J, Lamberghini F. Dental management in juvenile idiopathic arthritis. J Dent Child 2022;89(1):18–23.
5. Little JW, Miller CS, Rhodus NL. Little and Falace's Dental Management of the Medically Compromised Patient, Ninth Edition. Rheumatologic Disorders 2018;345–69.

A Patient Who Recently Underwent Total Temporomandibular Joint Replacement Reporting for Endodontic Therapy

Roopali Kulkarni, DMD, MPH*, Sunday Akintoye, BDS, DDS, MS

KEYWORDS

• Temporomandibular joint replacement • Total joint replacement • Endodontics

KEY POINTS

- Total joint replacement (TJR) of the temporomandibular joint (TMJ) is a surgical procedure completed when there is severe degeneration and dysfunction of the TMJ.
- Patients healing from TJR may have limitations in range of motion and experience TMJ-related pain.
- Patients with TMJ TJR may require shorter appointments, frequent breaks, and modifications during treatment such as using a bite block or mouth prop.

Medical Scenario: A 62-year-old male patient who recently underwent total TMJ replacement presents for evaluation and management of symptomatic #19. The patient had undergone total left alloplastic TMJ replacement surgery a month before initial presentation. His past medical history is significant for osteoarthritis. The patient had been previously diagnosed with severe TMJ degenerative joint disease, failed conservative treatments including physical therapy, pharmacologic management, appliance fabrication, and arthrocentesis. Before replacement, the patient underwent testing to rule out osteoporosis or osteopenia. A bone density scan revealed a T-score of greater than −1.0 with no fracture. Additionally, the patient underwent preoperative testing for allergy to the components of the metallic prosthesis, including cobalt chrome. The components included a titanium mandibular condyle and a polyethylene mandibular fossa implant. The patient had unremarkable healing after surgery but began to experience odontogenic pain.

Department of Oral Medicine, University of Pennsylvania School of Dental Medicine, Philadelphia, PA, USA
* Corresponding author. 240 South 40th Street, Room 215, Philadelphia, PA 19104.
E-mail address: RoopaliK@upenn.edu

Dent Clin N Am 67 (2023) 629–631
https://doi.org/10.1016/j.cden.2023.05.031

DENTAL MANAGEMENT DECISION AND JUSTIFICATION

A 62-year-old male patient presents to the dental clinic with a chief complaint of severe pain on the lower left side. He reports the pain began 2 weeks ago with no known precipitating factor. He describes the pain as a sharp pain that worsens with hot and cold foods. The pain is spontaneous and wakes the patient up at night. He took ibuprofen to ease the pain with some benefit.

His past medical history is significant for osteoarthritis. His medications include aspirin as needed for pain, and he has no known allergies. His surgical history is significant for total left alloplastic TMJ replacement surgery approximately 1 month before initial presentation. His family and social history is unremarkable. Pertinent positives in the review of systems included lower back pain and left knee pain.

Extraoral examination revealed mild swelling on the left side of the face and a palpable, nontender, mobile, less than 1 cm left submandibular lymph node. Examination of the temporomandibular joint revealed severe pain on palpation of the left preauricular area with a maximum intercuspal opening of 30 mm with moderate pain.

Limited intraoral examination revealed buccal swelling surrounding #19. #19 had a gross carious lesion with pulpal exposure. The patient's main priority was to eliminate pain and ultimately to save the tooth.

Due to the patient's goals, root canal therapy was initiated on the tooth. Although at this time controversial, the *American Academy of Orthopedic Surgeons* delineates appropriate use criteria for antibiotic usage before dental procedures. In this patient where manipulation of tissue may occur with rubber dam placement, no significant immunosuppression but with a joint replacement less than 1 year from procedure, antibiotics may be appropriate under the guidelines. In patients not allergic to penicillin, the standard prescription is amoxicillin 2 g taken 1 hour before dental procedure. If allergic to penicillin, the recommended alternatives may include azithromycin or clarithromycin 500 mg taken 1 hour before the dental procedure, under the updated guidelines. The patient was not allergic to penicillin drugs and took amoxicillin 2 g 1 hour before the appointment. During the procedure, a bite block was placed inside the mouth to alleviate pressure and allow for stable opening. Breaks were provided to the patient by removing the bite block, rubber dam still in place, to reduce pain. Given the patient's general bodily pain, support was provided to his back and knee with a pillow and towel, respectively. The patient's movement laterally was limited due to the hinged movements of the prosthesis. Unreasonable forces applied to restive range of motion could cause loosening and breakage of the screw. Therefore, pressure was not directly placed on the mandible.

HIGHLIGHTS AND ADDITIONAL CONSIDERATIONS

- TJR of the TMJ is typically initiated when conservative measures of treatment have failed and the temporomandibular joint disease is end-stage.[1]
- TMJ TJR can help improve patient's quality of life in terms of diet, mastication, speech, and social interactions.[1,2]
- Based on the *American Dental Association* guidelines, antibiotic prophylaxis is not typically recommended for patients with prosthetic joint implants before dental procedures.[3,4]
- Based on the guidelines from the *American Academy of Orthopedic Surgeons*, antibiotic prophylaxis may be considered in patients with prosthetic joint implants before dental procedures based on appropriate use criteria.[3]
- Limitations in the range of motion can pose challenges when providing care and performing dental procedures. Frequent breaks and shorter appointments are recommended.

- Holistic care involves interdisciplinary management postsurgery to improve the range of motion and function. Emphasizing oral hygiene postprocedure and nutrition counseling is important to maintain overall oral health.[5]

CLINICS CARE POINTS

- Shorter dental visits and frequent breaks may be needed in patients with TMJ TJRs.
- Interdisciplinary care with performing surgeon can aid in determining whether or not antibiotic prophylaxis is needed before dental procedures.
- Given limitations in mobility, mouth props/blocks can be used during dental procedures.

DISCLOSURE

The authors have no disclosures.

REFERENCES

1. Bhargava D, Neelakandan RS, Dalsingh V, et al. A three dimensional (3D) musculoskeletal finite element analysis of DARSN temporomandibular joint (TMJ) prosthesis for total unilateral alloplastic joint replacement. J Stomatol Oral Maxillofac Surg 2019;120(6):517–22.
2. Yoda T, Ogi N, Yoshitake H, et al. Clinical guidelines for total temporomandibular joint replacement. Jpn Dent Sci Rev 2020;56(1):77–83.
3. Mercuri LG, Psutka D. Perioperative, postoperative, and prophylactic use of antibiotics in alloplastic total temporomandibular joint replacement surgery: a survey and preliminary guidelines. J Oral Maxillofac Surg 2011;69(8):2106–11.
4. Antibiotic Prophylaxis Prior to Dental Procedures. Available at: https://www.ada.org/resources/research/science-and-research-institute/oral-health-topics/antibiotic-prophylaxis. Accessed September 20, 2022.
5. Wojczynska A, Gallo LM, Bredell M, et al. Alterations of mandibular movement patterns after total joint replacement: a case series of long-term outcomes in patients with total alloplastic temporomandibular joint reconstructions. Int J Oral Maxillofac Surg 2019;48(2):225–32.

A Young Adult Patient with Rheumatoid Disorder Presents for the Evaluation of Limited Mouth Opening

Sara N. Aldosary, BDS, Takako I. Tanaka, DDS, FDS RCSEd*

KEYWORDS

• Juvenile idiopathic arthritis • JIA • Trismus • Temporomandibular joint • TMJ
• Ankylosis

KEY POINTS

- Juvenile Idiopathic Arthritis (JIA) is the most common chronic inflammatory rheumatic condition of children causing short and long-term disability.
- The temporomandibular joint (TMJ) involvement of JIA is frequent and it has been reported to range from 11% to 87% of the cases.
- Patients with JIA affecting TMJ may manifest jaw pain, facial asymmetry, retrognathia, and/or trismus.
- Early recognition of JIA and multidisciplinary patient care is critical for time management and a better prognosis.

MEDICAL SCENARIO

A 20-year-old African male complained of progressively limited mouth opening for 3 years with bilateral intermittent stabbing jaw pain. He had been diagnosed with an unspecified rheumatoid disorder; however, the patient did not follow up with any medical providers due to relocation. He had no other significant medical history and did not take any medications. His family and social history were non-contributory. He was underweight primarily due to poor intake resulting from limited mouth opening. The extraoral examination was unremarkable except for retrognathia and marked trismus with a maximum inter-incisal opening of 15 mm. TMJ muscles were non-tender to palpation. Orthopantomogram revealed marked morphological changes of the condylar heads and no TMJ spaces.

Division of Oral Medicine, Department of Oral Medicine Penn Medicine, University of Pennsylvania School of Dental Medicine, 240 South 40th Street, Philadelphia, PA 19104, USA
* Corresponding author.
E-mail address: takakot@upenn.edu

Dent Clin N Am 67 (2023) 633–635
https://doi.org/10.1016/j.cden.2023.05.035
dental.theclinics.com

DENTAL MANAGEMENT DECISION AND JUSTIFICATION

The assessment was TMJ bony ankylosis secondary to JIA. The patient was referred to Oral & Maxillofacial Surgery (OMFS) and Rheumatology for further evaluation and management. A presurgical CT angiogram of the neck was ordered, which confirmed ankylosis of multiple joints including the bilateral TMJ and cervicothoracic facet joints. CBCT showed bilateral total TM joint ankylosis. Based on further imaging and laboratory studies, the final diagnosis of seronegative polyarticular Juvenile Idiopathic Arthritis was made. The patient was treated initially with Methotrexate 10 mg weekly and folic acid 1 mg daily by rheumatology. Later, the patient was treated surgically with total TM joint replacement and normal function of his TMJ as well as aesthetic improvement was achieved.

JIA is a heterogeneous group of diseases that includes all forms of arthritis of unknown etiology with onset before the age of 16 years.[1] JIA is the most common chronic inflammatory rheumatic condition of childhood causing short and long-term disability.[1] Its prevalence has been found to be about 1 per 1000 births in the Scandinavian countries, UK, and US.[1]

According to the International League Against Rheumatism (ILAR) classification, there are seven mutually exclusive categories of JIA exist among which polyarthritis (rheumatoid factor –negative) and oligoarthritis account for the majority.[2] Laboratory tests such as rheumatoid factor (RF), antinuclear antibodies (ANAs), and HLA–B27 can be useful in defining the specific JIA category.[2] HLA-27 and ANAs are typically associated with uveitis which is one of the most common extra-articular manifestations of JIA.[3]

TMJ involvement of JIA is frequent and it has been reported between 17% and 87%.[4] Abnormality of craniofacial growth caused by JIA results in significant functional and esthetic complications.[3] While unilateral TMJ involvement can present as facial asymmetry and maxillary canting· bilateral involvement of JIA can manifest retrognathia.[4] Conventional radiographic evaluations may show the mandibular ramus shortening and increased antegonial notching. MRI is useful to identify articular joint inflammation with expanding role in diagnosing, managing, and monitoring JIA.[2]

JIA treatment typically starts with scheduled nonsteroidal anti-inflammatory drugs (NSAIDs) and/or intra-articular corticosteroid injections. Disease-modifying Antirheumatic drugs (DMARDs) such as Methotrexate are the second-line therapeutic intervention.[2] The goal of pharmacotherapy in JIA is to rapidly reduce disease activity and lead to clinical remission. Physical therapy and/or occupational therapy were recommended for those at risk of functional limitations.[4] Surgical intervention is indicated in cases of bony ankylosis and facial asymmetry, which is recommended to be performed after skeletal maturity.

JIA substantially affects patient's quality of life. Collaborative efforts among various health care professionals are essential for the successful management of JIA.

CLINICS CARE POINTS

- Generally the onset of JIA is before the age of 16 years.
- MRI is the gold standard for the radiographic diagnosis JIA involving TMJ's although, images such as CT scans are also useful.
- In most cases of TMJ JIA the RF, ANAs, and HLA-B27 are used for categorizing the type of JIA.

- Although, dental treatment is not contraindicated in patient's with JIA, in acute stages where there is trismus, patients are more medically treated.

DISCLOSURE

All authors declare that they have no commercial or financial conflict of interest related to the material in this article and have received no funding for the preparation of this article.

REFERENCES

1. Ravelli A, Martini A. Juvenile idiopathic arthritis. Lancet 2007;369(9563):767–78.
2. Martini A, Lovell DJ, Albani S, et al. Juvenile idiopathic arthritis. Nat Rev Dis Primers 2022;8(1):5.
3. Rosenbaum JT, Dick AD. The Eyes Have it: A Rheumatologist's View of Uveitis. Arthritis Rheumatol 2018;70(10):1533–43.
4. Granquist EJ. Treatment of the Temporomandibular Joint in a Child with Juvenile Idiopathic Arthritis. Oral Maxillofac Surg Clin North Am 2018;30(1):97–107.

A Patient with Moderate-to-Severe Temporomandibular Joint Degenerative Joint Disease and Unilateral Joint Pain Presents for Oral Medicine Consult

Roopali Kulkarni, DMD, MPH*, Sunday Akintoye, BDS, DDS, MS

KEYWORDS

• Temporomandibular joint • Degenerative joint disease • Osteoarthritis

KEY POINTS

- Degenerative joint disease can affect the temporomandibular joint. In these circumstances, patients may experience pain or limitations in opening.
- Generalized osteoarthritis may also be present in the body. Pharmacologic management may include analgesics.
- Treatment of temporomandibular degenerative joint disease can include conservative treatments such as pharmacologic management with analgesics, physical therapy, and occlusal appliances. In rare occasions, surgical intervention may be required.
- Dental considerations include accurate diagnosis and subsequent management, potential modifications in chair positioning and supportive items such as towels or pillows to reduce stress on the body, shorter appointments, frequent breaks, and the use of dental bite blocks or mouth props during procedures to maintain opening and reduce pain.

Medical Scenario: A 76-year-old male patient with severe right-sided temporomandibular joint (TMJ) pain presents for consultation with oral medicine, referred by his general dentist. The patient had previously sought care with an oral and maxillofacial surgeon, who ordered an MRI of the temporomandibular joint and a computed tomography (CT) scan of the temporomandibular joint, at which point the diagnosis was severe bilateral TMJ degenerative joint disease (DJD). The patient was interested in seeking care with oral medicine.

DENTAL MANAGEMENT DECISION AND JUSTIFICATION

A 76-year-old male patient reports to the oral medicine clinic for evaluation of right-sided TMJ pain. The patient has had a 20+ year history of jaw pain. He describes

Department of Oral Medicine, University of Pennsylvania School of Dental Medicine, Philadelphia, PA, USA
* Corresponding author. 240 South 40th Street, Room 215, Philadelphia, PA 19104.
E-mail address: RoopaliK@upenn.edu

Dent Clin N Am 67 (2023) 637–639
https://doi.org/10.1016/j.cden.2023.05.032

the pain as a constant dull, ache on the left side with a sharper pain radiating to the ear on the right side. The sharper pain began 2 months ago after he bit into a sandwich. Stress, chewing, and opening wide make the pain worse. He has taken over-the-counter ibuprofen, acetaminophen, and was prescribed one course of methylprednisolone 4 mg (Medrol dosepak) per his dentist all with temporary benefit. He endorses headaches, right-sided ear ringing and pain, neck pain, and shoulder pain. He reports nighttime bruxism. He wears an occlusal guard that was fabricated by his dentist 5 years ago with benefit. He denies trauma to the head/neck region, denies any episodes of locked jaw, and denies history of orthodontic treatment.

His past medical history is significant osteoarthritis. His medications include ibuprofen. His allergies include fluconazole. He reports socially drinking alcohol and denies tobacco or recreational drug use. His surgical history is noncontributory. His family history is significant for hypertension. Review of systems was positive for generalized pain in the back, knees, and ankles.

The patient appeared to be a well-nourished, well-developed man in no apparent distress. Extraoral examination did not reveal lymphadenopathy, salivary gland enlargement, or thyromegaly. Cranial nerve examination II to XII were all grossly intact. Examination of the temporomandibular joint revealed pain on palpation of the right preauricular area and external auditory meatus. A bilateral reciprocal click was present with pain. The maximum intercuspal opening was 42 mm. There was no significant deviation or deflection noted. Lateral and protrusive movements were normal. On palpation of the masticatory and cervical muscles, moderate pain was noted on the anterior temporalis bilaterally, sternocleidomastoid bilaterally, left temporalis insertion, and left lateral pterygoid, and severe pain was noted on the right deep masseter, right temporalis insertion, and right lateral pterygoid.

Intraoral examination did not reveal gross caries, masses or ulcers but was notable for bilateral linea alba. A review of the previous panoramic radiograph, MRI, and CT were reviewed. Significant bilateral remodeling of the condylar head was noted in the panoramic radiograph. The CT revealed generalized sclerosis. Based on the history, physical examination, and radiographic findings, the diagnosis is consistent with articular disc disorder with reduction, myofascial pain of the muscles of mastication, and severe TMJ DJD.

The patient's goals were to avoid invasive treatment. A course of physical therapy for the jaw was prescribed. The patient's occlusal guard was evaluated and was deemed stable. Analgesics such as acetaminophen and ibuprofen were recommended on an as-needed basis. Additional recommendations included limiting jaw function by resting, avoiding excessive mouth opening, diet modifications, including avoiding hard, chewy, or crunchy foods, and heat/ice application.

HIGHLIGHTS AND ADDITIONAL CONSIDERATIONS

- Treatment of TMJ osteoarthritis (OA) consists of conservative therapies unless persistent or severe pain or dysfunction remains.[1–3]
  - Physical therapy may include the application of heat, ice, manual therapy, exercises, ultrasound, transcutaneous electrical nerve stimulation (TENS) stimulation, or other measures to reduce pain and increase function.
  - Pharmacologic management may include analgesics such as acetaminophen, aspirin, or ibuprofen. Muscle relaxants may aid in cases where muscle spasms or pain is present.
  - Occlusal appliances may aid in decreasing joint loading.
- CT of the TMJ is helpful to aid in diagnosing DJD.[3,4]

- Dental management considerations include shorter appointments, breaks during procedures to limit consistent mouth opening, and the use of bite blocks or mouth props to aid while performing procedures.
- General management requires interdisciplinary care, and dentists and specialists may be the first-line providers for diagnosis and treatment.[5]

CLINICS CARE POINTS

- TMJ DJD may be managed conservatively through occlusal appliances and pharmacologic management.
- For patients who fail conservative treatment, a surgical consultation may be warranted.
- Patients with TMJ DJD with pain may need shorter dental appointments and/or frequent breaks.

DISCLOSURE

The authors have no disclosures.

REFERENCES

1. Derwich M, Mitus-Kenig M, Pawlowska E. Interdisciplinary approach to the temporomandibular joint osteoarthritis-review of the literature. Medicina (Kaunas) 2020; 56(5):225.
2. Pantoja LLQ, Porto de Toledo I, Pupo YM, et al. Prevalence of degenerative joint disease of the temporomandibular joint: a systematic review. Clin Oral Investig 2019;23(5):2475–88.
3. Silva MAG, Pantoja LLQ, Dutra-Horstmann KL, et al. Prevalence of degenerative disease in temporomandibular disorder patients with disc displacement: A systematic review and meta-analysis. J Cranio-Maxillo-Fac Surg 2020;48(10):942–55.
4. Yap AU, Zhang Z, Cao Y, et al. Functional, physical and psychosocial impact of degenerative temporomandibular joint disease. J Oral Rehabil 2022;49(3):301–8.
5. Little JW, Miller CS, Rhodus NL. Rheumatologic Disorders. Little and Falace's Dental Management of the Medically Compromised Patient. Ninth Edition. p. 345–69.

A Patient with a Diagnosis of Gonococcal Arthritis and Symptomatic Bilateral Temporomandibular Joints Presents for Scaling and Root Planing

Roopali Kulkarni, DMD, MPH*, Sunday Akintoye, BDS, DDS, MS

KEYWORDS

• Gonococcal arthritis • Temporomandibular joint • Scaling and root planing

KEY POINTS

- Gonococcal arthritis is a rare complication of gonorrhea, which results in the inflammation of the joint from a bacterial infection.
- The TMJ can be impacted by gonococcal arthritis resulting in significant pain and reduction in function.
- With the increased risk of infection in scaling and root planing, active treatment of the condition is necessary.
- TMJ pain should be managed during the procedure with the segmental completion of the treatment, frequent breaks, and the use of dental bite blocks or mouth props to aid in mouth opening.

MEDICAL SCENARIO

A 17-year-old female patient with a diagnosis of gonococcal arthritis and bilateral temporomandibular joint disorder presents for scaling and root planing.

DENTAL MANAGEMENT DECISION AND JUSTIFICATION

A 17-year-old female patient presents to the dental clinic for scaling and root planing (SRP). The patient stated she has noticed swelling in her gums and bleeding after brushing. Upon initial evaluation, there was generalized plaque build-up and multiple

Department of Oral Medicine, University of Pennsylvania School of Dental Medicine, Philadelphia, PA, USA
* Corresponding author. 240 South 40th Street, Room 215, Philadelphia, PA 19104.
E-mail address: RoopaliK@upenn.edu

Dent Clin N Am 67 (2023) 641–643
https://doi.org/10.1016/j.cden.2023.05.034
0011-8532/23/

probing depths were >4 mm. Full-mouth series radiographs revealed generalized moderate horizontal bone loss. A comprehensive treatment plan was created based on the intraoral and radiographic findings.

At the time of SRP, the patient reported bilateral jaw joint pain and swelling. Her past medical history was non-contributory except for a diagnosis of gonorrhea. A review of systems revealed generalized joint pain in her knees and elbows. She thereafter reported a recent diagnosis of gonococcal arthritis, and the patient was advised to receive ceftriaxone via injection and a course of ibuprofen for pain management. An extraoral examination revealed bilateral moderate pain upon the palpation of the pre-auricular area and the bilateral masseter muscles.

Gonococcal arthritis can be a complication of gonorrhea, characterized by painful inflammation of joints due to transmission of *Neisseria gonorroheae*. Joints commonly involved in the condition include knees, ankles, wrists, and elbows. Typically, a complete blood count is obtained, where mild leukocytosis can be appreciated. Additionally, an erythrocyte sedimentation rate may be elevated in these patients. Imaging of affected joints may include an MRI or CBCT for the head and neck. Treatment typically involves antibiotics and analgesics. The treatment should involve addressing the underlying gonorrhea diagnosis, which is most commonly treated with ceftriaxone. Other possible antibiotics may include azithromycin or doxycycline. Analgesics may include non-steroid anti-inflammatories, or if more severe, short courses of corticosteroids. In this case, a panoramic image was obtained in order to evaluate for any radiographic changes of the jawbone. Mild condylar head flattening was noted bilaterally. The patient's primary goal was to eliminate the build-up on her teeth and reduce the bleeding of the gums.

With gonococcal arthritis not yet managed, the risk of infection and bleeding was noted and explained to the patient. With bilateral TMJ arthralgia and myalgia of the masseter muscles, the patient was advised that the dental treatment performed may exacerbate the pain symptoms. The patient understood and elected to proceed with treatment given their primary care goals. SRP was completed in segments per quadrant to avoid excessive bleeding and pain upon mouth opening. No risks were noted for local anesthesia administration. Given the bilateral jaw pain, one quadrant at a time was completed. The patient tolerated the procedure well over the course of multiple appointments. During the procedure, a bite block was used in order to increase opening and reduce pain upon active opening of the jaw.

The patient was then advised to rinse with Chlorhexidine 0.12% mouthwash twice daily for 2 weeks. Given the acute nature of the condition, the importance of systemic treatment of the gonococcal arthritis was emphasized to the patient. The patient noted improvement in their joint pain symptoms with the course of the ibuprofen. Conservative recommendations were provided to continue alleviating the muscular pain including the resting of the jaw, avoiding excessive mouth opening, avoiding hard, chewy, or crunchy foods, and moist-heat compresses.

HIGHLIGHTS AND ADDITIONAL CONSIDERATIONS

- Gonococcal arthritis is a type of septic arthritis which causes the inflammation of a joint due to a bacterial infection. It is a rare complication of those diagnosed with the sexually transmitted illness (STI) gonorrhea and is most commonly seen in sexually active female adolescents.[1,2]
- It can result in pain in bodily joints, including acute swelling and pain of the TMJ.[2–4]

- Given infection in the body, dental management should include conservative measures for disease control, education regarding possible sequelae of the disease, and recommendation of condition treatment with a referral.[5]
- During dental procedures, frequent breaks and shorter appointments are recommended to reduce stress on the TMJ.[5]

CLINICS CARE POINTS

- Patients with gonococcal arthritis need active treatment; therefore, interdisciplinary management is key.
- Patients with gonococcal arthritis with TMJ involvement may need shorter appointments and/or more frequent breaks.

DISCLOSURE

The authors have no disclosures.

REFERENCES

1. Al-Khalisy HM, Nikiforov I, Mansoora Q. Septic Arthritis in the Temporomandibular Joint. N Am J Med Sci 2015;7(10):480–2.
2. Bharmal RV, Chia M. Arthritis and dentistry. Primary Dental 2022;11(1):28–34.
3. Li R, Hatcher JD. *Gonococcal arthritis, StatPearls [Internet], . Treasure Island (FL).* StatPearls Publishing; 2022.
4. Mills F, Jadav P. Gonococcal arthritis. J Osteopath Med 2021;121(2):243.
5. Little JW, Miller CS, Rhodus NL. Rheumatologic Disorders. Little and Falace's Dental Management of the Medically Compromised Patient. Ninth Edition. St. Louis, MO: Elsevier; 2018. p. 345–69.

A Patient with a History of Fibromyalgia Reports for an Intraoral Incisional Biopsy

Roopali Kulkarni, DMD, MPH*, Sunday Akintoye, BDS, DDS, MS

KEYWORDS

- Fibromyalgia • Incisional biopsy • Lichenoid lesions

KEY POINTS

- Fibromyalgia, a chronic widespread pain syndrome, may cause idiopathic muscle pain and tenderness, fatigue, and sleep disturbances.
- Treatment of fibromyalgia includes both nonpharmacologic and pharmacologic therapies. Pharmacologic therapies may include tricyclic antidepressants, serotonin norepinephrine reuptake inhibitors, anticonvulsants, nonsteroidal anti-inflammatory drugs (NSAIDs), and muscle relaxants.
- Certain medications, such as NSAIDs, may result in lichenoid type lesions.
- Incisional oral biopsies of the lesions can help determine the precise diagnosis.
- Dental management of patients with fibromyalgia includes general recommendations, such as avoiding supine chair positioning, support for joints through pillows or towels, and shorter appointments. Specific recommendations for those undergoing incisional biopsies may include reducing the risk of bleeding by reviewing blood counts and using local hemostatic measures at the biopsy site.

MEDICAL SCENARIO

A 55-year-old female patient with a history of fibromyalgia presents for evaluation and biopsy of oral lesions, referred by her general dentist.

DENTAL MANAGEMENT DECISION AND JUSTIFICATION

A 55-year-old female patient presents to the oral medicine clinic for evaluation of oral lesions, referred by her general dentist. The patient has had a 5-year history of oral lesions with no known precipitating factor. The patient experiences mild pain and burning, which is worsened by spicy, acidic, and citrus foods. She has not tried

Department of Oral Medicine, University of Pennsylvania School of Dental Medicine, Philadelphia, PA, USA
* Corresponding author. 240 South 40th Street, Room 215, Philadelphia, PA 19104.
E-mail address: RoopaliK@upenn.edu

Dent Clin N Am 67 (2023) 645–647
https://doi.org/10.1016/j.cden.2023.06.002

anything to relieve the pain. In addition to the lesions, she endorses dry mouth, dry eyes, and difficulty swallowing. She denies any extraoral lesions.

Her past medical history is significant for fibromyalgia, hypertension, diabetes mellitus type 2, anxiety, and depression. Her medications include duloxetine, ibuprofen, lisinopril, and metformin. Her allergies include penicillin. She reports socially drinking alcohol and denies tobacco or recreational drug use. Her surgical history is noncontributory. Her family history is significant for hypertension, diabetes mellitus type 2, and history of cervical cancer. Review of systems was significant for loss of appetite, headaches, and neck and back pain.

The patient appeared to be a well-nourished, well-developed woman in no apparent distress. Extraoral examination did not reveal lymphadenopathy, salivary gland enlargement, or thyromegaly. Cranial nerve examination II–XII were all grossly intact. Intraoral examination did not reveal gross caries, masses, or ulcers but was notable for bilateral linea alba, generalized mild marginal gingival erythema, generalized plaque-buildup, moderate erythema, and Wickham striae in the bilateral buccal mucosa, most prominent in the left anterior buccal mucosa. Differential diagnosis included oral lichen planus or a lichenoid reaction. An incisional oral biopsy was planned for submission for hematoxylin-eosin staining and direct immunofluorescence staining. Given the patient's history of fibromyalgia, the patient was placed in a semisupine position during the procedure with neck support via a pillow. The patient was scheduled for a 2-week postoperative follow-up visit and was advised to follow up with their general dentist for routine cleanings.

HIGHLIGHTS AND ADDITIONAL CONSIDERATIONS

- Fibromyalgia, a chronic widespread pain syndrome,[1–3] may cause idiopathic muscle pain typically involving multiple regions of the body.[4,5] In a dental setting, patients may not feel comfortable receiving care in a supine position, depending on which muscles are involved.
- Support should be provided to the neck, back, and legs with pillows, towels, or other support devices. Shorter appointments should be scheduled to prevent excessive stress on the body.
- Some patients with fibromyalgia may take nonsteroidal anti-inflammatory drugs (NSAIDs) for pain management, which can result in prolonged bleeding. Proper local hemostatic measures during and after treatment are necessary.
- Lichenoid-type reactions may be present in patients with fibromyalgia who are on pharmacologic management with certain types of analgesics, like NSAIDs.[2,3]
- Patients with fibromyalgia may present with myofascial pain of the muscles of mastication.

CLINICS CARE POINTS

- Patients with fibromyalgia may need physical support throughout dental appointments.
- It is important to know what medications a patient with fibromyalgia is taking to manage the condition.
- Given that patients with fibromyalgia may have myofascial pain of the muscles of mastication, they may need mouth props or blocks used during dental treatment.

DISCLOSURE

The authors have no disclosures.

REFERENCES

1. Giorgi V, Sirotti S, Romano ME, et al. Fibromyalgia: one year in review 2022. Clin Exp Rheumatol 2022;40(6):1065–72.
2. Clauw DJ. Fibromyalgia: a clinical review. JAMA 2014;311(15):1547–55.
3. Maffei ME. Fibromyalgia: recent advances in diagnosis, classification, pharmacotherapy and alternative remedies. Int J Mol Sci 2022;21(21):7877.
4. Bair MJ, Krebs EE. Fibromyalgia. Ann Intern Med 2020;172(5):ITC33–48.
5. Sarzi-Puttini P, Giorgi V, Marotto D, et al. Fibromyalgia: an update on clinical characteristics, aetiopathogenesis and treatment. Nat Rev Rheumatol 2020;16(11): 645–60.

Scaling and Root Planning in a Patient Taking Chronic Corticosteroid Therapy for Lupus Erythematosus

Payam Mirfendereski, DDS[a], Rogan Magee, MD, PhD[b],
Katherine France, DMD, MBE[a,*]

KEYWORDS

• Systemic lupus erythematosus • Oral manifestations • Chronic corticosteroids
• Immunosuppression • Autoimmune disease

KEY POINTS

- Systemic lupus erythematosus (SLE) is a multisystem autoimmune disorder that can present with myriad oral manifestations.
- Medical management of SLE focuses on immunosuppression, and patients with SLE may be taking chronic systemic corticosteroid therapy.
- Chronic corticosteroid use has been associated with hypertension, hyperglycemia, osteoporosis, Cushing syndrome, and increased risk of opportunistic infection.
- Steroid supplementation is usually not indicated before or after non-surgical or surgical dental treatments in patients taking systemic oral corticosteroids.

MEDICAL SCENARIO

A 48-year-old female arrives for planned scaling and root planing of the maxillary and mandibular right quadrants. Her medical history is significant for systemic lupus erythematosus and hypertension. She is prescribed prednisone 7.5 mg and amlodipine 10 mg daily and acetaminophen 500 mg and tramadol 50 mg as needed for pain. She has not had a professional dental cleaning in 5 years due to dental anxiety. After being seated, she reports a heightened stress level over the week preceding her appointment. She also notes progressively worsening generalized gingival soreness and a burning sensation on the roof of her mouth and lower lip.

[a] Department of Oral Medicine, University of Pennsylvania School of Dental Medicine, 240 South 40th Street, Philadelphia, PA 19104, USA; [b] Department of Neurology, Penn Medicine, 3400 Spruce Street, Philadelphia, PA 19104, USA
* Corresponding author.
E-mail address: kfrance@upenn.edu

Dent Clin N Am 67 (2023) 649–651
https://doi.org/10.1016/j.cden.2023.05.018
dental.theclinics.com

DENTAL MANAGEMENT DECISION AND JUSTIFICATION

Dentists should be familiar with the orofacial manifestations of systemic lupus erythematosus (SLE). Precautions with and consequences of chronic oral corticosteroid therapy should also be considered. SLE is a multisystem autoimmune disease with strong female predominance and prevalence of 241:100,000 in North America.[1] SLE is diagnosed based on clinical and serologic findings. Oral lesions are included in the standard diagnostic criteria.[2] Musculoskeletal, cutaneous, cardiovascular, pulmonary, renal, and ocular involvement are also possible in SLE.[1]

The classic oral mucosal lesion seen in SLE consists of an erythematous discoid lesion with white keratotic striae in the periphery. Oral ulcers, white plaques, telangiectasias, and petechiae are also commonly identified.[3] While the hard palate is most often affected, the buccal and labial mucosae are also commonly affected. Desquamative gingivitis has also been associated with SLE. Oral lesions in SLE often mirror those seen in oral lichen planus and can be associated with mucosal burning, soreness, or sensitivity, which at times complicates compliance with oral hygiene.[1]

Systemic therapies for SLE focus on immunosuppression. Hydroxychloroquine remains one of the mainstays of management.[4] Oral systemic corticosteroid therapy for SLE is well-established, in higher doses for acute symptomatic flares and lower doses for maintenance therapy. Cyclophosphamide, methotrexate, azathioprine, and mycophenolate mofetil represent alternative steroid-sparing therapies. Recently, biologics such as rituximab and belimumab have been employed in the treatment of recalcitrant disease.[3]

Symptomatic inflammatory oral lesions of SLE that remain unresponsive to systemic therapy may be managed with moderate- to high-potency topical corticosteroids, including solutions for disseminated lesions and gels for focal lesions.

Both the underlying inflammatory pathophysiology of SLE and the effects of maintenance corticosteroids are associated with an increased risk of periodontitis.[5,6] Dry mouth is also common in SLE, leading to decreased pH and greater plaque and calculus accumulation.[1] More frequent hygiene maintenance should therefore be considered for these patients.

In addition to an increased predisposition to periodontitis, chronic oral corticosteroid use is associated with myriad adverse effects that further complicate periodontal and dental management. Maintenance corticosteroid use is associated with hypertension, hyperglycemia, osteoporosis, and Cushing syndrome.[7] Significantly, chronic corticosteroid use increases the risk of opportunistic infection.

Dentists should pay special attention to SLE-associated nephritis. For pain management after scaling and root planing, non-steroidal anti-inflammatory drugs must be used with caution given potential nephrotoxicity.[1] Acetaminophen should be preferentially recommended (**Table 1**). Dentists should also be aware of the possibility of comorbid antiphospholipid antibody syndrome and the increased risk of post-procedural bleeding that chronic anticoagulation may confer.[4]

Table 1
Medications frequently prescribed in dentistry to avoid in patients with systemic lupus erythematosus and renal dysfunction, plus recommended alternatives

Medications Frequently Used in Dentistry that Have Predominantly Kidney-Dependent Elimination	Recommended Alternatives
NSAIDs, acetylsalicylic acid	Acetaminophen
Penicillins, cephalosporins, tetracyclines	Clindamycin, azithromycin

Supplemental corticosteroid dosing prior to dental procedures in at-risk patients has been historically controversial. It is broadly understood that major surgical procedures and certain comorbidities may warrant steroid supplementation due to the associated physiologic stress and resultant increased cortisol demand. Maintenance dosing of prednisone for patients with SLE is recommended at less than or equal to 7.5 mg/d, with the complete withdrawal of steroids as soon as possible.[4] This dose ranges below the 10 mg/d threshold often employed for steroid supplementation before major surgeries. Further, more recent assessments such as those made by Little and Falace and others indicate no need for steroid supplementation before or after surgical and non-surgical dental procedures.[7] Proper stress management protocols, effective anesthesia, and atraumatic techniques remain paramount.

CLINICS CARE POINTS

- Patients with systemic lupus erythematosus (SLE) may present with oral lesions secondary to their disease, as well as involvement of various organs.
- Patients may be taking chronic corticosteroids, which can put them at risk of opportunistic infections and other systemic complications.
- Routine supplementation of small doses of corticosteroids for dental treatment is no longer recommended.

CONFLICT OF INTEREST

All authors declare that they have no commercial or financial conflict of interest related to the material in this article and have received no funding for the preparation of this article.

REFERENCES

1. Benli M, Batool F, Stutz C, et al. Orofacial Manifestations and Dental Management of Systemic Lupus Erythematosus: A Review. Oral Dis 2021;27(2):151–67.
2. Aringer M, Costenbader K, Daikh D, et al. European League Against Rheumatism/American College of Rheumatology Classification Criteria for Systemic Lupus Erythematosus. Ann Rheum Dis 2019;78(9):1151–9.
3. Mays JW, Sarmadi M, Moutsopoulos NM. Oral Manifestations of Systemic Autoimmune and Inflammatory Diseases: Diagnosis and Clinical Management. J Evid Based Dent Pract 2012;12(3 Suppl):265–82.
4. Fanouriakis A, Kostopoulou M, Alunno A, et al. Update of the EULAR Recommendations for the Management of Systemic Lupus Erythematosus. Ann Rheum Dis 2019;78:736–45.
5. Hussain SB, Leira Y, Zehra SA, et al. Periodontitis and Systemic Lupus Erythematosus: A Systematic Review and Meta-Analysis. J Periodontal Res 2022;57(1):1–10.
6. Brasil-Oliveira R, Cruz ÁA, Sarmento VA, et al. Corticosteroid Use and Periodontal Disease: A Systematic Review. Eur J Dermatol 2020;14(3):496–501.
7. Chan MH. Update on Management of the Oral and Maxillofacial Surgery Patient on Corticosteroids. Oral Maxillofac Surg Clin North Am 2022;34(1):115–26.

A Female Patient Recently Diagnosed with Sjogren Syndrome Presents to the Dental Office Seeking Upper and Lower Complete Dentures

Irene H. Kim, DMD, MPH[a], Purvi C. Patel, DMD[b], Mel Mupparapu, DMD, MDS, Dipl. ABOMR[a,*]

KEYWORDS

- Sjogren syndrome • Xerostomia • Xerophthalmia • Sicca syndrome

KEY POINTS

- Sjogren syndrome (SS) is a chronic, systemic autoimmune condition that leads to the destruction of exocrine glandular epithelium resulting in symptoms of xerostomia and xerophthalmia.
- Oral manifestations of SS include higher risk of dental caries, gingivitis, friable mucosa, candidiasis, angular cheilitis, and enlarged salivary glands.
- The treatment of SS is generally palliative and supportive, targeting relief of symptoms and prevention.
- Dentists should be aware of the oral manifestations of SS to help their patients manage their xerostomia and achieve a better quality of life.

MEDICAL SCENARIO

A 57-year-old woman in no apparent distress presented to the clinic for the evaluation of full maxillary and mandibular dentures. She complained of difficulty wearing her current dentures and a generalized dryness in her mouth, throat, and eyes. The dryness in her mouth also made it difficult to eat. Her medical history was significant for rheumatoid arthritis (RA) and a recent diagnosis of secondary Sjogren syndrome (SS) 6 months ago. Intraoral examination revealed that the patient was fully edentulous with little salivary pooling. The mucosa appeared friable, and the tongue was fissured. Extraoral

[a] Department of Oral Medicine, University of Pennsylvania School of Dental Medicine, Philadelphia, PA, USA; [b] New York University College of Dentistry, New York, NY, USA
* Corresponding author. Department of Oral Medicine, Penn Dental Medicine, 240 South 40th Street, Philadelphia, PA 19104.
E-mail address: mmd@upenn.edu

Dent Clin N Am 67 (2023) 653–656
https://doi.org/10.1016/j.cden.2023.05.019
0011-8532/23/

examination revealed redness around the eyes and slight swelling of the parotid glands. The dryness in the mouth and eyes was consistent with Sicca syndrome (SiS). Her current prostheses were in fair condition and attempts to adjust the denture were unsuccessful.

DENTAL MANAGEMENT DECISION AND JUSTIFICATION

The patient was referred to the Department of Periodontics for treatment planning implants. Due to the xerostomia and RA, a fixed or semifixed prosthesis was recommended. As SS progresses, the lack of saliva will hinder the retention of the dentures and may increase the likelihood of intraoral traumatic lesions from the removable prostheses. As the associated RA progresses, the ability of the patient to insert and remove the prostheses may become more difficult. To help the patient manage their current SS symptoms, the patient was given instructions to help alleviate SiS such as carrying a water bottle to lubricate the oral mucosa and using lip balms and creams to manage dry skin. Emphasis was also placed on maintaining routine dental visits so that the dentist can monitor any other oral manifestations such as candidiasis and angular cheilitis. In addition, routine medical visits were encouraged to manage the associated RA.

SS is a common autoimmune disease that is chronic and systemic and can exist as primary SS (pSS) or secondary SS. It is considered secondary when SS is associated with other autoimmune diseases such as RA, systemic lupus erythematosus, systemic sclerosis, and primary biliary cirrhosis.[1] There are approximately 4 million people in the United States who have SS with a reported female to male ratio of 9:1 and peaks of incidence around the age of 30 and 50 years.[1,2] SS is a disease that is associated with the immune-mediated destruction of epithelia of the exocrine glands, in particular the salivary and lacrimal glands. As a result, patients commonly present with SiS, which consists of xerophthalmia and xerostomia.[2] Other glandular systems that may be affected include the skin (xeroderma, eyelid dermatitis), nasal passages, and vagina. Patients may also present with extraglandular symptoms such as fatigue, myalgia, arthralgia, depression, and anxiety.[2]

The diagnosis of SS in a previously unsuspected case can be especially challenging because the symptoms are nonspecific, and SiS may not be present at the time of diagnosis. If a patient is in the dental chair with symptoms suggestive of SS, then a full panel of investigations is mandated before continuing dental treatment. A diagnosis of pSS is confirmed on positive results for the following tests: salivary gland biopsy, ultrasound, and anti-Sjögren-syndrome-related antigen A auto antibodies (Ro/SSA) serology as well as an unstimulated whole saliva flow rate value less than or equal to 0.1 mL/min and a Schirmer's test value less than or equal to 5 mm/min.[3] Management of SS often requires a multidisciplinary approach involving specialists (**Box 1**). There is no cure for SS, and the management of SS is palliative. Patients are encouraged to limit alcohol, smoking, and environments that are dry to prevent the exacerbation of SiS. Frequent drinking or rinsing with water and the use of lubricants are also recommended. Muscarinic agonists such as pilocarpine hydrochloride can serve as sialagogues to improve xerostomia but these agents can also cause unwanted diaphoresis.[4]

Due to the immune-mediated destruction of salivary glands, dentists should be aware of the oral manifestations of SS. These include friable mucosa, fissured tongue, plaque accumulation, gingivitis, unusual caries presentation (root, cervical, incisal), infections such as candidiasis, enlarged salivary glands, traumatic oral lesions, and challenges with removable oral prostheses. In terms of management of the dental

Box 1
Summary of diagnosis, oral manifestations and dental management of patients with Sjogren Syndrome

SS diagnosis

- There is no one test to diagnose, involves careful review of all symptoms with specialists (rheumatologist, ophthalmologist, dentist)
- Tests can include the following:
  - Blood and urine test for presence of common antibodies found in SS
  - Antinuclear antibody test to determine autoimmune disorder
  - Schirmer's test for tear production
  - Lip biopsy to test for type and severity of inflammation
  - Salivary gland imaging, salivary gland function tests

Common oral manifestations primarily due to xerostomia

- Friable and dry mucosa
- Fissured tongue
- Root, cervical, incisal caries
- Candidiasis
- Enlarged salivary glands
- Traumatic oral lesions

Dental management

- Frequent hydration
- Discontinuation of medications known to cause xerostomia
- Topical fluoride treatments, fluoride varnish applications, glass ionomer restorations
- Patient education on diet and hygiene, routine dental visits
- Implants preferred over removable prostheses

This table summarizes the diagnosis, oral manifestations, and dental management of Sjogren syndrome.

SS patient, the lack of the protective properties of saliva puts patients at very high risk for dental caries. Topical fluoride treatments are highly recommended. Caries management can also be reinforced with patient education on diet and minimally invasive procedures such as fluoride varnish application and glass ionomer restorations.[5] Edentulous and partially edentulous patients have difficulty with removable prostheses because of their dry and friable oral mucosa. Dental implants have been reported to have a low failure rate of 4.1% in SS patients and may be a good option in these cases.[6]

SS in dental patients present unique challenges mainly due to the associated xerostomia. Dentists should be aware of the symptoms to work closely and patiently in treating and managing their patients to improve their quality of life as best as possible.

CLINICS CARE POINTS

- Sjogren Syndrome is a common autoimmune disease that can exist as primary or secondary (associated with other autoimmune disorders such as Lupus, scleroderma, Rheumatoid arthritis etc).
- The diagnosis of SS is confirmed positively via salivary gland biopsy, ultrasound and anti-Ro/SSA serology.
- SS in dental patient can bring about challenges related to treatment due to associated xerostomia as it increases the risk for caries. Topical fluoride treatments are highly recommended.
- Pilocarpine hydrochloride can be used as sialagogue to improve xerostomia.

DISCLOSURE

Nothing to disclose.

REFERENCES

1. Vivino FB, Bunya VY, Massaro-Giordano G, et al. Sjogren's syndrome: An update on disease pathogenesis, clinical manifestations and treatment. Clin Immunol 2019;203:81–121.
2. Generali E, Costanzo A, Mainetti C, et al. Cutaneous and Mucosal Manifestations of Sjogren's Syndrome. Clin Rev Allergy Immunol 2017;53(3):357–70.
3. Van Ginkel MS, Glaudemans AWJM, van der Vegt B, et al. Imaging in Primary Sjögren's Syndrome. J Clin Med 2020;9(8):2492.
4. Mariette X, Criswell LA. Primary Sjogren's Syndrome. N Engl J Med 2018;378(10): 931–9.
5. Young DA, Frostad-Thomas A, Gold J, et al. Secondary Sjogren syndrome: A case report using silver diamine fluoride and glass ionomer cement. J Am Dent Assoc 2018;149(8):731–41.
6. Chrcanovic BR, Kisch J, Wennerberg A. Dental implants in patients with Sjogren's syndrome: a case series and a systematic review. Int J Oral Maxillofac Surg 2019; 48(9):1250–9.

A Patient with a History of Multiple Myeloma Presents for the Evaluation of Oral Lesion and Burning Sensation of the Mouth

Irene H. Kim, DMD, MPH[a], Walter W. Hong, MD, Dip.ABPN[b], Sophia Oak, BS[c], Brad M. Hong, BA[a], Mel Mupparapu, DMD, MDS, Dipl.ABOMR[a,*]

KEYWORDS

• Multiple myeloma • Plasma cell dyscrasia • Blood dyscrasia • Bisphosphonate • Zoledronic acid • Bone marrow transplant • Chemotherapy • Oral manifestations

KEY POINTS

- Multiple myeloma (MM) is a malignant disease of plasma cells. Patients with MM commonly present with anemia, bone pain, fatigue, and weight loss. In addition to medical history and clinical examination, the diagnostic work-up for MM comprises of laboratory tests and radiographic examinations to detect bone changes.
- Common oral manifestations of MM include bony lesions in the mandible and maxilla that can present as painful bony swellings, epulis formation, or teeth mobility.
- Patients with MM treated with antiresorptive medications, such as bisphosphonates and denosumab, are at high risk of developing osteonecrosis of the jaw.
- Achieving optimal hemostasis can be a challenge in patients with MM due to risk of thrombocytopenia and platelet dysfunction. Patients may also be susceptible to infection due to myelosuppression of the bone marrow.
- A multidisciplinary approach is required to manage people with MM. Dental assessment prior to starting antiresorptive medication is crucial.

MEDICAL SCENARIO

A 65-yr-old Caucasian female presents to the admissions clinic at the Dental School seeking comprehensive dental care. She was diagnosed with multiple myeloma about

[a] Department of Oral Medicine, University of Pennsylvania School of Dental Medicine, Philadelphia, PA, USA; [b] Replimune, Clinical Development, Woburn, MA, USA; [c] Temple University Kornberg School of Dentistry, Philadelphia, PA, USA
* Corresponding author. Department of Oral Medicine, University of Pennsylvania School of Dental Medicine, 240 South 40th Street, Philadelphia, PA 19104.
E-mail address: mmd@upenn.edu

Dent Clin N Am 67 (2023) 657–661
https://doi.org/10.1016/j.cden.2023.05.014
dental.theclinics.com

a decade ago and went through several treatment protocols that included bone marrow transplant, chemotherapy and use of corticosteroids. She is stable now and had a referral from her oncologist for dental treatment. Her oncologist mentioned that the patient received several doses of zoledronic acid 4 mg intravenously every 3-4 weeks during her active treatment for multiple myeloma and currently stopped since her remission.

Dental Management Decision and Justification

Prior to any dental procedures, the patient's oncologist was consulted to review her medical history and laboratory values. During the first visit, oral-hygiene instructions were strongly reinforced because of the patient's history of bisphosphonates and the increased risk for osteonecrosis of the jaw. Laboratory values, especially the platelet and neutrophil counts, were requested from her treating physician. In treatment plans requiring invasive dental procedures, laboratory blood values of platelet counts >50,000 platelets/μL and neutrophil counts >1,000/mm^3 are necessary to achieve proper hemostasis and prevent infection. The patient did not have any neck or back pain at the time of visit, but care was taken in patient positioning to accommodate the patient and make her comfortable. The patient was also told to feel free to take breaks if she felt fatigued.

Multiple myeloma (MM) is a hematologic malignancy belonging to a class of disorders known as plasma cell dyscrasias. It is a clonal plasma cell proliferative disorder characterized by an abnormal increase in monoclonal immunoglobulins. The overproduction of plasma cells can lead to end-organ damage resulting in destructive bone lesions (**Fig. 1**), renal injury, and abnormal laboratory values such as anemia and

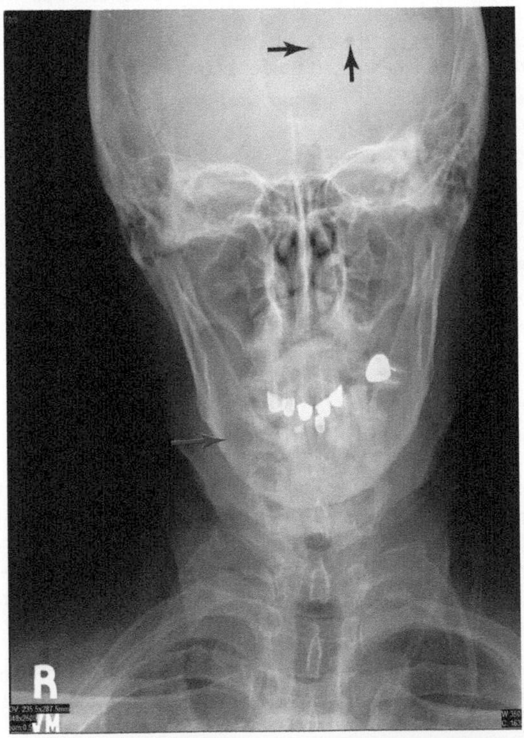

Fig. 1. Reverse Town view skull radiograph of a patient with multiple myeloma. Black arrows points to multiple myeloma lesions in the skull. The red arrow points to a large osteolytic area in the right mandible consistent with a localized lesion, Plasmacytoma.

Box 1
Summary of dental issues in patients with multiple myeloma

Medications
- Anti-resorptive (such as bisphosphonates)
  - Increased risk of osteonecrosis of the jaw.
  - Need to work closely with oral surgeon and medical team to coordinate treatment planning.
- Corticosteroids
  - Adrenal insufficiency resulting from high-dose steroidal therapy used to treat patients with MM.
  - Dental practitioners need to work closely with the medical team to determine if there is a need for supplemental steroids in select dental procedures such as extractions.

Treatment considerations
- Bleeding
  - Hemostasis may be difficult due to thrombocytopenia, platelet dysfunction, and hyperviscosity.
  - Dental practitioners need to consult with the medical team to determine blood values.
  - Invasive dental procedures should not be performed when platelet counts <50,000 platelets/μL.
- Infection
  - Patients with MM are susceptible to infections due to myelosuppression in the bone marrow.
  - Dental practitioners need to consult the medical team to determine laboratory values.
  - Invasive dental procedures should not be performed when neutrophil values < 1,000/mm^3.
- Conscious sedation and general anesthesia
  - Conscious sedation and general anesthesia can be used to reduce anxiety in patients with MM.
  - Dental practitioners must monitor hemoglobin levels and must not consider these options if hemoglobin is < 10 g/dL.
  - Transfusions may be necessary if the patient is anemic.
- Timing of dental treatment
  - MM-related symptoms such as anemia and mouth ulcers limit the patients' ability to tolerate dental treatment.
  - Short, morning appointments are recommended to minimize fatigue.
- Patient position
  - Patients with MM often experience neck and back pain.
  - Pillow or neck rest may help alleviate pressure on the back.
  - Patients may need to take breaks during treatment.

hypercalcemia.[1] MM is the second most common hematologic malignancy in the United States. An estimated 34,470 cases will be diagnosed with MM, resulting in 12,640 deaths in 2022.[2] It is more common among men than women, and most frequently affects people over the age of 65. There is a higher prevalence of MM reported in the Black/African American population.[3]

The diagnosis of MM requires specific clinical features. These features include evidence of 10% or more clonal plasma cells in the bone marrow or a plasmocytoma proven by biopsy, and evidence of end-organ damage such as hypercalcemia, renal insufficiency, anemia, or bone lesions.[1] Once a diagnosis is made, further studies can aid in determining the prognosis and staging of the disease. These include fluorescent in situ hybridization to detect high-risk cytogenic abnormalities, serum β_2 microglobulin, and lactate dehydrogenase.[2]

Patients with MM are treated by a multidisciplinary team led by a hematologist specializing in myeloma, with goals of stabilizing the progression of the disease and treating related symptoms such as bone pain, anemia, renal damage and hypercalcemia.[3] First-line induction therapy involves a combination of an injectable proteasome inhibitor such as bortezomib, and an oral immunomodulatory agents such as lenalidomide and dexamethasone. For eligible patients, induction therapy combined with an autologous hematopoetic stem cell transplant followed by maintenance lenalidomide is the standard of care.[1] Treatment is dependent upon the age and fitness of the patient, as well as the staging of the disease. Of note to dental practitioners is the use of bisphosphonates such as pamidronate and zoledronic acid during chemotherapy, and in patients with MM who are asymptomatic.

Common oral maxillofacial manifestations of MM are bony lesions in the mandible and maxilla that can clinically present as pain, bony swelling, epulis formation, or sudden teeth movement.[4] A classic radiographic appearance is punched-out lesions unrelated to teeth apices and skull lesions with ill-defined borders.[3] Dental considerations for the treatment of patients with MM are related to their medications and laboratory values. These considerations include the use of bisphosphonates and corticosteroids, bleeding, and infection, as summarized in **Box 1**.

MM is a complex plasma-cell disorder characterized by multiple end-organ damage. As a result, there are many factors that the dental practitioner should consider in treating patients with MM. Dentists should be aware of these factors to provide optimal care for patients with MM and prevent potential complications such as infection and bleeding, which can occur with some of the more invasive dental procedures. Working closely with a multidisciplinary team that takes into consideration laboratory blood values, medications, and the symptoms of MM are essential in the dental treatment of patients with MM.

CLINICS CARE POINTS

- Achieving optimal hemostasis can be a challenge in patients with MM due to the risk of thrombocytopenia and platelet dysfunction. Reviewing medical history and laboratory values in conjunction with the patient's oncologist or hematologist is prudent prior to any dental procedures.
- In treatment plans requiring invasive dental procedures, laboratory blood values of platelet counts >50,000 platelets/μL and neutrophil counts >1,000/mm^3 are necessary to achieve proper hemostasis and prevent infection.
- Patients with MM may present with anemia. Dental practitioners should arrange appointments at suitable times for the patient, who may not be able to tolerate long appointments due to fatigue.
- For patients who experience neck and back pain, careful positioning of the dental chair is necessary to avoid pressure to the back. It is important to allow time for rest during treatment as needed.
- Bisphosphonate introduces a high risk of osteonecrosis of the jaw, so preventive dental care is imperative. Oral-hygiene instructions should be emphasized in the early phase of treatment.

DISCLOSURE

Nothing to disclose.

REFERENCES

1. Cowan AJ, Green DJ, Kwok M, et al. Diagnosis and management of multiple myeloma: a review. JAMA 2022;327(5):464–77.

2. Mikhael J, Bhutani M, Cole CE. Multiple myeloma for the primary care provider: a practical review to promote earlier diagnosis among diverse populations. Am J Med 2023;136(1):33–41.
3. Abed HH, Al-Sahafi EN. The role of dental care providers in the management of patients prescribed bisphosphonates: brief clinical guidance. Gen Dent 2018; 66(3):18–24.
4. Borggrefe J, Giravent S, Campbell G, et al. Association of osteolytic lesions, bone mineral loss and trabecular sclerosis with prevalent vertebral fractures in patients with multiple myeloma. Eur J Radiol 2015;84(11):2269–74.

A Patient Undergoing Treatment of Hematologic Malignancy Reports for Oral Evaluation

Payam Mirfendereski, DDS[a], Katherine France, DMD, MBE[a,*]

KEYWORDS

• Acute myeloid leukemia • Oral manifestations • Leukemic gingival infiltration
• Chemotherapy • Opportunistic infection

KEY POINTS

- Acute myeloid leukemia (AML) is an aggressive hematologic malignancy that carries a poor prognosis.
- Oral lesions associated with AML include gingival bleeding, gingival hyperplasia, mucosal ulcers, and petechiae.
- Chemotherapy for AML and other hematologic malignancies has been associated with numerous oral complications, including mucositis, bleeding, xerostomia, opportunistic infections, dental pain, and neurological issues.

MEDICAL SCENARIO

A 68-year-old man presents to the dental clinic for an examination with a chief complaint of gingival inflammation. He reports that his gums bleed frequently with eating and brushing, and he thinks he may need a deep cleaning. He also reports an intermittent metallic taste in his mouth that coincides with recurrent white patches on his dorsal tongue. He endorses persistent red, dry, and itchy labial commissures as well. His medical history is significant only for acute myeloid leukemia (AML). He has recently completed induction therapy with a 10-day course of cytarabine plus daunorubicin and at the time of examination is undergoing consolidation therapy with 4 cycles of high-dose cytarabine.

DENTAL MANAGEMENT DECISION AND JUSTIFICATION

Oral lesions are often the first clinical presentation of AML, and their identification by the dental provider may play a critical role in the ultimate diagnosis of the condition.

[a] Department of Oral Medicine, University of Pennsylvania School of Dental Medicine, 240 South 40th Street, Philadelphia, PA 19104, USA
* Corresponding author.
E-mail address: kfrance@upenn.edu

Dent Clin N Am 67 (2023) 663–665
https://doi.org/10.1016/j.cden.2023.05.016

AML is an aggressive hematologic malignancy marked by the proliferation of myeloid blasts that fail to undergo normal differentiation. The annual incidence of AML in the United States rests greater than 20,000. The disease is most common in adults older than 65 years but affects children to a lesser extent as well.[1] AML has a markedly poor prognosis, with a 5-year survival rate of 28.3%.[1] The prognosis for AML has improved over the past decades thanks to new drug therapies, with 5-year survival directly dependent on aggressive treatment. The low overall rate reflects cases of late diagnosis, inability to tolerate treatment, and lower remission rates among older patients with AML. Formal diagnosis of AML requires a peripheral blood sample or a bone marrow biopsy. AML is classified is based on a combination of immunophenotypic, morphologic, and genetic factors.[2]

Before diagnosis, patients with AML may present with nonspecific systemic complaints such as fatigue, fever, pallor, persistent or recurrent infections, and ecchymoses or petechiae on the skin and mucosa.[3] However, oral lesions may be the patient's principal complaint, highlighting the importance of the dental professional being aware of the oral manifestations of AML for early referral to a medical specialist. The most common oral manifestations of AML are gingival bleeding, gingival hyperplasia, mucosal ulcers, and petechiae.[2] Leukemic gingival infiltration may be responsible in part for the gingival symptoms, whereas thrombocytopenia, immunodeficiency, and secondary inflammatory infiltration are also thought to contribute.[3] In the patient mentioned earlier, leukemic gingival infiltration and thrombocytopenia could account for the predisposition to bleeding with eating and brushing. Although less common than soft tissue involvement, oral hard tissues can also be affected in AML, presenting as osteolytic lesions or progressive tooth mobility with no local cause.[3]

If left untreated, AML can be fatal within weeks to months.[2] Management of AML has traditionally involved induction chemotherapy followed by consolidation therapy after initial remission. Standard chemotherapy for AML is comprised of the combination of cytarabine and an anthracycline.[1] Hematopoietic stem cell transplantation remains an option for patients at high risk for recurrence of disease. Numerous targeted therapies are also being studied and used for certain subgroups of patients with AML.[1] Chemotherapy and select target therapies have been associated with numerous oral complications, including mucositis, bleeding, xerostomia, opportunistic infections, dental pain, and neurological issues.[4] The aforementioned patient's complaints regarding metallic taste, recurrent white patches on the tongue, and erythematous labial commissures may reflect an opportunistic candida infection.

Dental evaluation and treatment of the patient with AML should be coordinated with the patient's oncologist. Considerations for dental treatment are determined by whether the patient presents before, during, or after chemotherapy. Before chemotherapy, the goal of the dentist should be to evaluate the patient, educate them on the oral complications of chemotherapy, and treat their dental needs in accordance with their medical status. Active sources of infection should be eliminated to the extent feasible given that chemotherapy can cause myelosuppression that predisposes patients to opportunistic infections. Myelosuppression induced by chemotherapy usually peaks 2 weeks postinitiation, and dental intervention during this time should be limited to truly emergent needs and remain as minimally invasive as possible.[5] The timing between cycles of chemotherapy should also be considered when planning dental treatment with interventions preferentially timed during relative hematological stability. Gingival hyperplasia associated with AML has been shown to regress within 1 month of initiation of chemotherapy.[2] Daily oral hygiene is critical in reducing secondary gingival inflammation, and rinsing twice daily with 0.12% chlorhexidine gluconate has been shown to be effective toward this purpose.[4] If any dental treatment is to be performed, antibiotic prophylaxis should be administered in patients with an absolute neutrophil count less than 500/μL and considered in patients with counts less than 1000/μL.[5] Patients undergoing more intensive chemotherapy regimens may also be placed on antifungal or antiviral prophylaxis during chemotherapy, and any signs of opportunistic infections such as intraoral candidiasis, angular cheilitis, or recurrent herpes simplex or varicella zoster virus infections should be treated as appropriate in concert with the patient's oncology team. Oral mucositis due to chemotherapy can be managed in accordance with the most current clinical practice guidelines.[6] After chemotherapy, the patient may continue to experience complications such as xerostomia, dysgeusia, or neuropathies, which should be evaluated for and managed as appropriate.

CLINICS CARE POINTS

- Acute myeloid leukemia (AML) can commonly present with oral soft tissue involvement and may also cause bone lesions
- Prompt diagnosis and treatment of AML are essential for patient recovery
- Patients with AML are at higher risk of opportunistic infections, including oral viral, fungal, and bacterial infections

CONFLICT OF INTEREST

All authors declare that they have no commercial or financial conflict of interest related to the material in this article and have received no funding for the preparation of this article.

REFERENCES

1. Newell LF, Cook RJ. Advances in acute myeloid leukemia. BMJ 2021;375:n2026.
2. Quispe RA, Aguiar EM, de Oliveira CT, et al. Oral manifestations of leukemia as part of early diagnosis. Hematol Transfus Cell Ther 2022;44(3):392–401.
3. Cammarata-Scalisi F, Girardi K, Strocchio L, et al. Oral Manifestations and Complications in Childhood Acute Myeloid Leukemia. Cancers 2020;12(6):1634.
4. Wong HM. Oral complications and management strategies for patients undergoing cancer therapy. Sci World J 2014;2014:581795.
5. Zimmermann C, Meurer MI, Grando LJ, et al. Dental treatment in patients with leukemia. J Oncol 2015;2015:571739.
6. Elad S, Cheng KKF, Lalla RV, et al. MASCC/ISOO clinical practice guidelines for the management of mucositis secondary to cancer therapy. Cancer 2020;126(19):4423–31 [published correction appears in Cancer. 2021 Oct 1;127(19):3700].

A Patient Presenting for Dental Extraction After Completion of Chemotherapy

Walter W. Hong, MD, Dip. ABPN[a], Irene H. Kim, DMD, MPH[b], Brad M. Hong, BA[b], Sophia Oak, BS[c], Mel Mupparapu, DMD, MDS, Dipl. ABOMR[b,*]

KEYWORDS

- Acute myeloid leukemia • Acute granulocytic leukemia • Chemotherapy
- Radiation therapy • Hematopoetic stem-cell transplant • Graft-versus-host disease
- Dental abscess • Oral manifestations

KEY POINTS

- Acute myeloid leukemia (AML), the most common type of acute leukemia in adults, results from the abnormal proliferation and differentiation of myeloid stem cells in the bone marrow.
- Oral manifestations of AML include gingival hyperplasia, pale mucosa, poor wound healing, petechiae, ecchymoses, candidiasis, recurrent herpes infection, and ulcerations in the oral mucosa.
- The first-line AML treatment is chemotherapy. The most common complication of high-dose chemotherapy is mucositis. Additional treatments for AML include radiation therapy and hematopoetic stem-cell transplant (HSCT).
- When treating patients with AML, dental practitioners should carefully monitor hematological indices before performing dental procedures. All the preventive and curative oral measures should be carried out with the consultation of hematologist or oncologist.

MEDICAL SCENARIO

A 75-year-old White man presents to the admissions clinic at the Dental School seeking care for his abscessed mandibular tooth (tooth # 30). He was diagnosed with acute myeloid leukemia (AML) 1 year ago. Patient started the chemotherapy under the guidance of his oncologist at the hospital. The chemotherapy was completed a week ago when the patient started to notice pain and swelling in relation to tooth #30 and was

[a] Replimune, Clinical Development, Woburn, MA, USA; [b] Department of Oral Medicine, University of Pennsylvania School of Dental Medicine, Philadelphia, PA, USA; [c] Temple University Kornberg School of Dentistry, Philadelphia, PA, USA
* Corresponding author. Department of Oral Medicine, Penn Dental Medicine, 240 South 40th Street, Philadelphia, PA 19104.
E-mail address: mmd@upenn.edu

Dent Clin N Am 67 (2023) 667–670
https://doi.org/10.1016/j.cden.2023.05.020
0011-8532/23/

Abbreviations	
AML	Acute Myeloid leukemia
HSCT	hematopoetic stem-cell transplant
GVHD	graft-versus-host disease

referred to the dental clinic by his treating oncologist. Patient was weak and was brought into the dental clinic for an emergency visit. Intraoral examination revealed a large occlusal carious lesion in relation to tooth # 30. Patient had an earlier composite restoration that was fractured and, in its place, had secondary caries. Patient also had a swelling around the buccal gingiva in the region of #30; a small draining sinus was noted, which discharged pus on expression. The general oral health of the patient was not very good, and he wanted help. An intraoral radiograph showed a large apical rarefying osteitis in relation to the mesial root of #30. The tooth tested nonvital.

DENTAL MANAGEMENT DECISION AND JUSTIFICATION

AML is a malignant disease that results from the abnormal proliferation and differentiation of myeloid stem cells in the bone marrow.[1] It is the most common form of acute leukemia seen in adults, with an estimated 21,450 new AML cases diagnosed in 2019. It has a slightly higher prevalence among men over women, with a median age at diagnosis of approximately 68 years old.[2] The estimated number of deaths attributed to AML in 2019 is nearly 11,000, which is approximately 1.8% of all cancer deaths in the United States.[3]

The signs and symptoms of AML include fatigue, dyspnea, bruising, bleeding, and infections, sometimes involving the brain, skin, and gingiva. AML can progress rapidly and is typically fatal within weeks or months if left untreated.[2] The diagnosis is based on bone-marrow aspiration and clinical laboratory values.[3]

The first-line treatment of AML is chemotherapy with the goal of inducing remission. The 1970s discovery of the activity of cytarabine (ara-C) and of anthracyclines in AML, and the combination of them into the "3 + 7 regimen" (3 days of daunorubicin + 7 days of cytarabine), has long been considered the standard of care, resulting in long-term cures of 30% to 40% among younger patients with AML. Earlier studies focused on patients aged 50 to 55 year and reported 5-year survival rates of 40% to 45%. Later studies including patients aged up to 60 years reported 5-year survival rates of 30% to 35%. These intensive chemotherapy regimens are applied commonly in older patients (aged 60 years and older) and result in 5-year survival rates of less than 10% to 15%.[4]

The 3 phases of chemotherapy are induction, consolidation, and maintenance. Consolidation is achieved via several forms of treatment, usually with higher dose cytarabine or with a combination of cytarabine and idarubicin, daunorubicin, or mitoxantrone.[5] Oncologists achieve maintenance therapy via oral chemotherapy with drugs such as azacytidine or via continuation of the targeted drug that was part of their initial treatment.[5]

Additional treatments available include other forms of chemotherapy, radiation therapy, hematopoietic stem-cell transplant (HSCT). The common oral manifestations[6] are summarized in **Box 1**. Patients who qualify for a stem cell transplant may receive HSCT. When a patient receives HSCT, a major complication is graft-versus-host disease (GVHD). In GVHD, the host rejects the graft and immunocompetent donor cells attack the patient's antigens, leading to a decrease in T lymphocytes. Oral manifestations of GVHD are lichen-like features, hyperkeratotic plaques, mucoceles, and

Box 1
Summary of dental issues in patients with acute myeloid leukemia

Oral Manifestations

- First signs
  - Gingival hyperplasia caused by leukemic infiltration in oral tissues.
  - Periapical inflammatory lesions, clinically and radiographically, caused by leukemic infiltration.
  - Pale mucosa, poor wound healing, petechiae, ecchymoses
  - Candidiasis, herpes infections, ulcerations
- During treatment
  - Most common manifestation is mucositis
  - Bleeding, increased rate of dental caries, infection, abscesses
  - Herpetic stomatitis, candidiasis
  - Salivary gland dysfunction, xerostomia, dysgeusia, pain
- Undergoing HSCT
  - Lichen-type features, hyperkeratotic plaques, fibrosis with limited mouth opening due to long-term immunosuppression and GVHD
  - Higher likelihood of developing malignancies such as squamous cell carcinoma

Treatment considerations

- Noninvasive dental procedures may be performed at any stage of treatment
- Invasive dental procedures involving higher risks of hemostasis and infection require consultation with the medical team to evaluate blood laboratory values
- Hematological indices to monitor for invasive dental procedures:
  - Invasive dental procedures should not be performed when platelet counts less than 50,000 platelets/μL
  - Invasive dental procedures should not be performed when neutrophil values less than $1000/mm^3$
- Other considerations
  - Antibiotic coverage when neutrophil counts are less than $1000/mm^3$
  - In acute cases with high risk, patients may need to be treated in a hospital setting where blood transfusions can be administered.

fibrosis limiting mouth opening. These patients are also at a higher risk of developing squamous cell carcinoma.[7] Invasive dental procedures should not be performed when platelet counts are less than 50,000 platelets/μL and neutrophil counts are less than $1000/mm^3$. Antibiotic prophylaxis is usually recommended when neutrophil counts are less than $1000/mm^3$. The treatment assessments before dental procedures are summarized in **Box 1**.

CLINICS CARE POINTS

- When treating patients with AML, dental practitioners should carefully monitor hematological indices before performing dental procedures. All the preventive and curative oral measures should be carried out with the consultation of hematologist or oncologist.
- Invasive dental procedures should not be performed when platelet counts are less than 50,000 platelets/μL and neutrophil counts are less than $1000/mm^3$. Antibiotic prophylaxis is also usually recommended when neutrophil counts are less than $1000/mm^3$.
- At the completion of all planned courses of chemotherapy, close monitoring of the patient is required until all oral side effects of therapy have resolved.

DISCLOSURE

Nothing to disclose.

REFERENCES

1. De Kouchkovsky I, Abdul-Hay M. Acute myeloid leukemia: a comprehensive review and 2016 update. Blood Cancer J 2016;6(7):e441.
2. Siegel RL, Miller KD, Jemal A. Cancer statistics. CA Cancer J Clin 2019; 69(1):7–34.
3. Nix NM, Price A. Acute Myeloid Leukemia: An Ever-Changing Disease. J Adv Pract Oncol 2019;10(Suppl 4):4–8.
4. Kantarjian H, Kadia T, DiNardo C, et al. Acute myeloid leukemia: current progress and future directions. Blood Cancer J 2021;11(2):41.
5. American Cancer Society. Typical Treatment of Acute Myeloid Leukemia. Available at: https://www.cancer.org/cancer/acute-myeloid-leukemia/treating/typical-treatment-of-aml.html. Accessed April 23, 2023.
6. Cammarata-Scalisi F, Girardi K, Strocchio L, et al. Oral Manifestations and Complications in Childhood Acute Myeloid Leukemia. Cancers 2020;12(6):1634.
7. Zimmermann C, Meurer MI, Grando LJ, et al. Dental treatment in patients with leukemia. JAMA Oncol 2015;2015:571739.

A 65-Year-Old Man with Recent History of Radiation Therapy to the Head and Neck Reporting for Treatment of a Non-restorable Tooth

Payam Mirfendereski, DDS[a], Jacob W. Trotter, MD[b],
Katherine France, DMD, MBE[a,*]

KEYWORDS

- Head and neck radiation • Intensity-modulated radiation therapy
- Nonrestorable tooth • Dental restorability • Ferrule effect • Root canal therapy
- Extraction • Osteoradionecrosis

KEY POINTS

- Head and neck radiation confers an elevated risk for osteonecrosis after dental surgery through the triad of bony hypovascularity, hypocellularity, and hypoxia.
- Intensity-modulated radiation therapy (IMRT) and proton therapy have allowed for improved sparing of areas unaffected by disease and reduced the rates of dental complications after radiation.
- Osteoradionecrosis remains of particular concern at radiation doses above 60 Gy.
- Dental restorability is influenced by the tooth's structural integrity, periodontal status, and patient factors.
- Conservative nonsurgical treatments such as endodontic therapy may be advisable for nonrestorable teeth in cases where osteoradionecrosis is of concern.

MEDICAL SCENARIO

A 65-year-old man arrives to the dental clinic with a nonrestorable right lower molar. His medical history is notable for a history of squamous cell carcinoma of the left tongue involving the left mandible diagnosed 3 years earlier. For this diagnosis, he underwent left partial glossectomy and left partial mandibulectomy followed by adjuvant

[a] Department of Oral Medicine, University of Pennsylvania School of Dental Medicine, 240 South 40th Street, Philadelphia, PA 19104, USA; [b] Department of Radiation Oncology, Penn Medicine, 3400 Civic Center Boulevard, Philadelphia, PA 19104, USA
* Corresponding author.
E-mail address: kfrance@upenn.edu

Dent Clin N Am 67 (2023) 671–674
https://doi.org/10.1016/j.cden.2023.05.021
dental.theclinics.com
0011-8532/23/

radiation therapy to the left oral cavity and bilateral neck lymph nodes (**Fig. 1**). Since radiation, he has experienced moderate xerostomia. He has been using oral fluoride dental paste but has not followed-up with his dentist since his preradiation cleaning and evaluation. He has never smoked. On general examination, the patient is alert and oriented. Vitals are within normal limits. Complete head and neck examination shows mild fibrosis of the bilateral neck and mild limitation of opening. Intraoral examination reveals a partially edentulous mandible, a coronal fracture on tooth #30 at the gingival margin, and diminished salivary flow from the submandibular glands. Radiographs reveal a 5-mm periapical radiolucency associated with #30.

DENTAL MANAGEMENT DECISION AND JUSTIFICATION

Following radiation treatment of cancers of the head and neck, patients are at an increased risk of complications following extractions or other major dental procedures. Risks include poor wound healing and osteoradionecrosis with the areas of the molar and premolar teeth of the mandible at greatest risk. In recent years, advanced radiation techniques such as intensity-modulated radiation therapy (IMRT) or proton therapy have allowed for improved radiation sparing of the unaffected areas with decreased rates of dental complications. However, even with these techniques, tumor location, size, and other factors may create a need for substantial radiation to be delivered to uninvolved areas such as the contralateral teeth or mandible. These uninvolved areas can see anywhere from full dose to minimal dose, which can greatly affect the individual's risk profile for complications. For this reason, it is recommended that dental providers review the patient's radiation records and, if possible, speak with the patient's radiation oncologist to understand the treatment fields and identify the areas that are at an increased risk of dental complications when treating patients with earlier radiation to the head and/or neck.

When treatment planning for the patient with a history of head and neck radiation, the dentist should pay special attention to maximizing tooth restorability. Tooth restorability is complex and multifaceted, and structural integrity is only one of the main determinants. The ferrule effect has been established as a traditional requisite for structural integrity, with a 360° collar comprising at least 2 mm of healthy tooth structure above the alveolar ridge usually considered the threshold for an acceptable

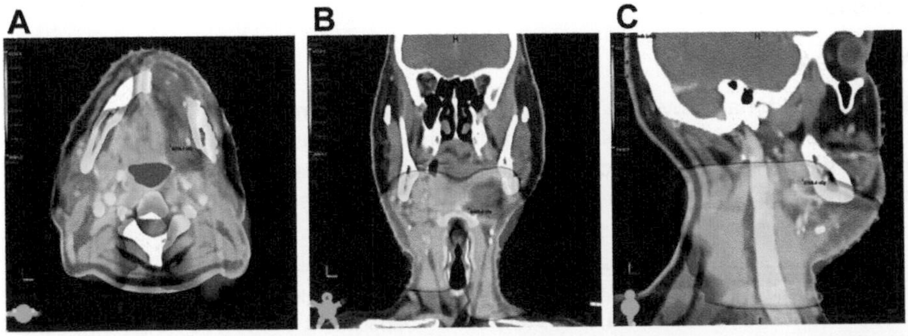

Fig. 1. Radiation dose distributions of a patient undergoing IMRT as adjuvant treatment of a squamous cell carcinoma of his left tongue. The patient was prescribed 60 Gy to the left resection bed and 54 Gy to the bilateral neck nodal basins. In this patient, the ipsilateral mandible received a maximum dose of 65 Gy (placing this patient at increased concern for complication after dental extraction) and the contralateral mandible received a max of 52 Gy. Mean dose to the mandible was 32 Gy. (*A*) Axial, (*B*) coronal, and (*C*) sagittal.

restorative prognosis.[1] Periodontal factors such as crown to root ratio, clinical attachment loss, and mobility are also closely linked to tooth restorability. Restorability can also be influenced by patient factors such as oral hygiene compliance.

Although extraction tends to be the recommended treatment of a clinically nonrestorable tooth, patients with a history of head and neck radiation must be evaluated carefully for the viability of this option due to the possible risk for delayed healing and osteonecrosis of the jaw. Osteoradionecrosis is the result of radiation-induced bony hypovascularity, hypocellularity, and hypoxia, and extractions can result in osteonecrosis by causing soft tissue trauma and bone exposure. Osteoradionecrosis is of particular concern at radiation doses above 60 Gy.[2] In the current medical scenario, as illustrated in **Fig. 1**, the patient received approximately 52 Gy to the right mandible in the area of #30. Although this is less than 60 Gy, it still conveys an elevated risk that should be considered in creating the treatment plan, including by salvaging this and other teeth wherever possible.

Root canal therapy with coronectomy followed by primary gingival closure over the remaining root(s) can be performed as a palliative treatment of an otherwise nonrestorable tooth. Although root canal therapy can effectively resolve root infections, bone fill tends to be slower in the irradiated patient.[2] Rubber dam isolation must be carefully used in these patients to avoid impingement and trauma to soft tissues. Trismus, another potential complication of head and neck radiation, can complicate both rubber dam placement and the use of endodontic instrumentation in the posterior mandible. During obturation, it is important to avoid endodontic overfill as well as thermal damage to the periodontal ligament given the expected delayed healing in irradiated tissues. Chlorhexidine rinses are recommended before and after treatment because this can help reduce the possibility of bacteremia associated with soft tissue trauma.[3]

If all attempts to save the nonrestorable tooth prove ineffective and extraction must be performed, technique and timeframe should be carefully considered. It has been recommended that extractions be preferentially performed within 6 months postradiation therapy because irradiated tissue fibroses progressively with time.[2] Extractions should be performed with minimal trauma to soft tissues, with any indicated alveoloplasty, and with tension-free primary closure. Certain medical regimens, such as hyperbaric oxygen therapy, pentoxifylline and tocopherol with or without clodronate, and antibiotics have been used to prevent or manage osteoradionecrosis in cases of unavoidable extractions.[4,5] However, definitive benefit from any of these regimens remains to be established.

CLINICS CARE POINTS

- Patients with histories of head and neck radiation to the oral cavity and surrounding structures are at increased risk of developing osteoradionecrosis.
- Nonrestorable teeth in such patients can be considered for any restorative treatments that allow the tooth to be saved, such as root canal therapy.
- Exact dosages of radiation to various structures must be considered in treatment planning these patients.

CONFLICT OF INTEREST

All authors declare that they have no commercial or financial conflict of interest related to the material in this article and have received no funding for the preparation of this article.

REFERENCES

1. Esteves H, Correia A, Araújo F. Classification of Extensively Damaged Teeth to Evaluate Prognosis. J Can Dent Assoc 2011;77:b105.
2. DeLaura T, Caughey J, Kufta K, et al. Considerations for Dental Management of Post-Radiation Head and Neck Cancer Patients: A Literature-Based Critical Review. Sel Read Oral Maxillofac Surg 2020;27:4.
3. Farmakis ETR, Merzioti M. Endodontic Treatment and Prevention of Osteonecrosis in Patients undergoing Radiation and/or Bisphosphonate Therapy: A review of the Literature and Recommended Treatment Protocol. MedP Dent Sci 2022;1(1): mpds–202202001.
4. Banjar A, Patel V, Abed H. Pentoxifylline and Tocopherol (Vitamin E) with/without Clodronate for the Management of Osteoradionecrosis: A Scoping Review. Oral Dis 2021. https://doi.org/10.1111/odi.14058.
5. Beech N, Robinson S, Porceddu S, et al. Dental Management of Patients Irradiated for Head and Neck Cancer. Aust Dent J 2014;59(1):20–8.

A Patient with a History of Tonsillar Cancer Presents for Evaluation of Exposed Alveolar Bone in the Mouth

Takako I. Tanaka, DDS, FDS, RCSEd[a,*], Rabie Shanti, DMD, MD[b]

KEYWORDS

- Osteoradionecrosis • Oral cancer • Head and neck cancer • Hyperbaric oxygen
- Radiotherapy • Smoking

KEY POINTS

- Osteoradionecrosis (ORN) may manifest as prolonged exposed bone without pain after many years of radiation therapy for head and neck cancer.
- Early recognition of ORN by thorough oral examination is essential because of potential radial jaw resection required as a treatment.
- Timely and appropriate referrals to the experts are warranted for successful management of ORN.

MEDICAL SCENARIO

A 49-year-old man was referred to the oral medicine clinic for evaluation of "exposed bone" along the right mandible that has been present for about 1 year. The patient denies associated pain or change in size of the area of concern; however, he endorsed mild right lower lip numbness. Patient expressed his concerns about prolonged bone exposure. The patient's past medical history was significant for right tonsillar squamous cell carcinoma treated by chemoradiation 10 years prior and subsequent marginal mandibulectomy 1 year ago. He denies facial swelling nor drainage from the lesion. Extraoral examination was unremarkable. Intraoral examination revealed a small 3 $\times$ 2 mm oval-shaped exposed bone with mild erythema in the surrounding area on the posterior lower right alveolar ridge.

[a] University of Pennsylvania School of Dental Medicine; [b] University of Rutgers School of Dental Medicine
* Corresponding author.
E-mail address: takakot@upenn.edu

Dent Clin N Am 67 (2023) 675–677
https://doi.org/10.1016/j.cden.2023.06.003
0011-8532/23/

DENTAL MANAGEMENT DECISION AND JUSTIFICATION

Clinical impression was osteoradionecrosis (ORN). A 0.12% chlorhexidine oral suspension was prescribed to the patient to use twice daily to control the local infection and a maxillofacial computed tomography image was obtained to determine the extent of the lesion. Because of chronic bone exposure, the patient was subsequently referred to oral and maxillofacial surgery for further evaluation and management. During irrigation, bone spicule was detached from the right posterior mandible. The spicule was sent for histologic evaluation, which revealed necrotic bone. Contemporaneously, the diagnosis of ORN of the jaw was confirmed. After counselling the patient regarding treatment plan, the patient received hyperbaric oxygen therapy followed by further surgical debridement and local tissue rearrangement of right mandible.

ORN is a late adverse effect of radiation therapy because of poor vascularity of the irradiated area of the bone. ORN is more commonly seen in patients with head and neck malignancy who received more than 6000 cGy of radiation. It occurs in approximately 2% of patients receiving 6000 cGy to 7000 cGy ionizing radiation and 9% of patients who receive more than 7000 cGy.[1] ORN may occur long after radiation therapy. Newer radiation techniques, such as intensity-modulated radiation therapy, have a lower incidence of ORN.[2]

ORN commonly affects the mandible, particularly the area with thin mucosal coverage, such as mylohyoid ridge or mandibular tori. Patient may not experience pain; however, prolonged exposed bone can result in chronic infection, and further develop swelling, osteomyelitis, or cutaneous fistulae.

Of note, thorough examination including palpation of the cervical lymph node evaluation is critical. The timing and dose of radiation should be obtained from the radiation oncologist and chemotherapy and imaging (eg, radiographs, panoramic images, computed tomography, MRI) should be reviewed.

ORN treatment often requires a multidisciplinary approach including oral medicine, oral and maxillofacial surgery, radiology, and hyperbaric medicine specialists.

Primary managements of ORN include saline irrigations, antibiotics (during the infection), gentle sequestrectomy, and treatment with hyperbaric oxygen.[2–5] Radical surgery including resection of the jawbone with reconstruction is necessary for persistent and extensive ORN. Meticulous oral hygiene measures and periodic oral evaluations may prevent or reduce the incidence of ORN. Because ORN can severely impact patients' quality of life, research should be continued to further ameliorate this serious adverse effect of radiation therapy.

CLINICS CARE POINTS

- ORN is a late adverse effect of radiation therapy, which is more commonly seen in patients with head and neck malignancy who received more than 6000 cGy of radiation.
- ORN commonly affects the mandible, particularly areas with thin mucosal coverage, such as the mylohyoid ridge or mandibular tori.
- The use of hyperbaric oxygen may be considered to prevent or treat ORN; however, a case-by-case assessment is recommended because of the lack of consistent data on its effectiveness.

DISCLOSURE

None.

REFERENCES

1. Davis DD, Hanley ME, Cooper JS. Osteoradionecrosis. Treasure Island (FL): StatPearls Publishing; 2022. StatPearls.
2. Tanaka TI, Chan HL, Tindle DI, et al. Updated clinical considerations for dental implant therapy in irradiated head and neck cancer patients. J Prosthodont 2013;22(6):432–8. https://doi.org/10.1111/jopr.12028.
3. Lang K, Held T, Meixner E, et al. Frequency of osteoradionecrosis of the lower jaw after radiotherapy of oral cancer patients correlated with dosimetric parameters and other risk factors. Head Face Med 2022;18(1):7.
4. Möring MM, Mast H, Wolvius EB, et al. Osteoradionecrosis after postoperative radiotherapy for oral cavity cancer: a retrospective cohort study. Oral Oncol 2022;133:106056.
5. Forner LE, Dieleman FJ, Shaw RJ, et al. Hyperbaric oxygen treatment of mandibular osteoradionecrosis: combined data from the two randomized clinical trials DAHANCA-21 and NWHHT2009-1. Radiother Oncol 2022;166:137–44.

A Patient Presents for Dental Extraction and Goes into Sickle Cell Crisis in the Dental Chair

Walter W. Hong, MD, Dipl. ABPN[a], Irene H. Kim, DMD, MPH[b],
Adeyinka F. Dayo, BDS, DMD, MS[b],
Mel Mupparapu, DMD, MDS, Dipl. ABOMR[b,*]

KEYWORDS

- Sickle cell disease (SCD) • Hemoglobin S • Vaso-occlusive pain • Dental
- Sickle cell crisis

KEY POINTS

- Sickle Cell Disease is a multisystem disorder caused by a genetically variant hemoglobin.
- The defective HbS assumes a sickle shape and the resulting RBC stasis in the capillaries leads to ischemia and pain.
- Severe pain crisis managed by multiple medications including narcotics and non-steroidal anti-inflammatory agents.
- Oral manifestations of SCD include mucosal pallor, yellow tissue coloration, radiographic abnormalities, delayed tooth eruption, disorders of the enamel and dental mineralization and mental nerve neuropathy.
- Dentists should be knowledgeable about SCD, where early intervention and anxiety management are essential in their care.

MEDICAL SCENARIO

A 21-yr-old male patient in no apparent distress presented to the dental clinic complaining of pain in relation to posterior teeth in the lower left jaw. The medical history was significant for sickle cell disease (SCD) managed by his primary care physician. His medications included low-dose oral morphine 15 mg/12 hours for acute episodes of vaso-occlusive pain, and up to150 mg daily for chronic pain. Extraoral examination was within normal limits. Intraoral examination revealed a restored mandibular right left second M, restorations in teeth 2, 14, 15 as well. Fair to poor

[a] Replimune, Clinical Development, Woburn, MA, USA; [b] Department of Oral Medicine, University of Pennsylvania School of Dental Medicine, Philadelphia, PA, USA
* Corresponding author. Department of Oral Medicine, University of Pennsylvania, School of Dental Medicine, 240 South 40th Street, Philadelphia, PA 19104.
E-mail address: mmd@upenn.edu

Dent Clin N Am 67 (2023) 679–682
https://doi.org/10.1016/j.cden.2023.05.015 dental.theclinics.com
0011-8532/23/

oral hygiene, moderate generalized plaque accumulation, gingivitis, and a yellowish coloration of the buccal and labial mucosae were noted. Radiographic examination revealed large mesio-occlusal restoration on #18 with an associated mild widening of PDL space on the mesial root apex on a panoramic radiograph. The Lamina dura was intact. The treatment plan was to replace the restoration in tooth # 18 under local anesthesia. At this point, the patient became very anxious. Prior to the administration of local anesthesia, the patient started complaining about generalized body aches with leg pain and within a matter of minutes was in intolerable pain.

DENTAL MANAGEMENT DECISION AND JUSTIFICATION

The patient was escalating to a hemolytic crisis. Per emergency protocol, the attending called 911 to manage the sickle cell crisis. The patient was comfortable before his visit and did not take his low-dose morphine, and when he became very anxious during his visit, he went into sickle cell crisis. All dental procedures were halted and the patient was managed by the emergency medical team.

SCD is an inherited autosomal recessive hemoglobinopathy caused by the single amino acid substitution of valine for glutamic acid in the beta-chain leading to a defective hemoglobin S (HbS). The pathology of HbS is characterized by the formation of long chains of hemoglobin when it is deoxygenated within the capillary beds distorting the red blood cell (RBC) into a sickle shape. The abnormal sickle cells have increased adhesion to endothelial walls and hemolyze quickly leading to a compensatory increase in the production of reticulocytes. This sickling and hemolytic action initiates an inflammatory reaction involving the endothelium, white blood cells, and platelets. RBC hemolysis and sickling, along with endovascular inflammation cause acute and chronic organ damage at the cellular level. The acute pain that patients experience is caused by the vaso-occlusion and its associated ischemia.[1] The criterion for diagnosing an SCD pain crisis is a patient report of pain. Severe crises are commonly managed with parenteral opioids and nonsteroidal anti-inflammatory drugs.[2]

Common medical complications of this multiorgan disease include acute chest syndrome, acute ischemic stroke, splenic sequestration, leg ulcerations, renal failure, and hepatopathy among many others.[3] The most common oral manifestation of SCD is mucosal pallor and yellow tissue coloration which is a consequence of the chronic hyperbilirubinemia and hemolytic anemia caused by the RBC destruction. Other oral manifestations include radiographic abnormalities, delayed tooth eruption, disorders of the enamel and dental mineralization and mental nerve neuropathy.[4]

Worldwide, there are approximately 300,000 infants born with SCD each year, with more than half living in sub-Saharan Africa and India. There are approximately 100,000 individuals with SCD who live in the United States.[2] In the United States, newborn screening is performed on all infants while in other countries it is optional. Hemoglobin variants can be detected in blood samples from heel sticks using high-performance liquid chromatography or isoelectric focusing, and the diagnosis can be confirmed with hemoglobin electrophoresis.[2]

Patients with SCD presenting to a dental office should be examined carefully to rule out any current infections, neurologic deficits, or other organ involvement before formulating a dental treatment plan to avoid prolonged and complicated procedures. Dentists should work closely with the patient's hematologist and primary care physician to manage the SCD. Oftentimes patients neglect their dental needs because of the multiple health issues that arise from SCD and patients tend to prioritize their medical problems over any dental issues. As a result, SCD dental patients often present as an emergency when they are in severe dental pain.[4] Recommendations for the dental

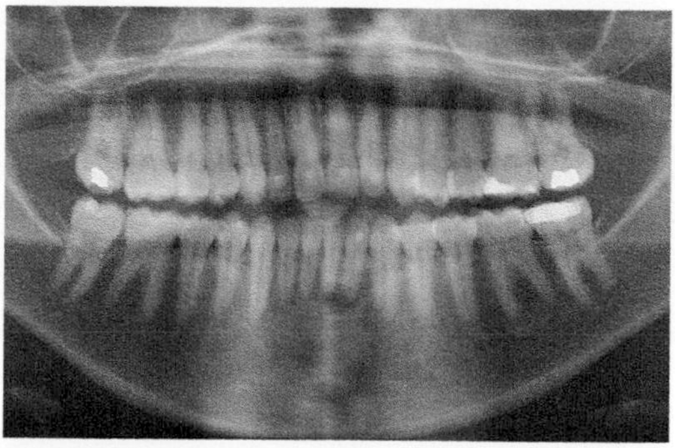

Fig. 1. Panoramic radiograph showing altered trabeculation and enlarged bone marrow spaces suggestive of increased demand for oxygenation. Although many patients with SCD may not exhibit this degree of variation of trabeculation, it is to be expected especially if they have SCD and not a sickle cell trait.

treatment of patients with SCD include preventive care and anxiety management.[4] Routine dental visits and early intervention will reduce or eliminate emergency visits. This will also reduce dental anxiety as the patient becomes more familiar with the dental environment and does not associate the experience with the more invasive procedures associated with emergency care. Other strategies to decrease dental anxiety may involve the use of anxiolytics and sedatives.[4] Radiographic changes may include enlarged bone marrow spaces and sparse trabeculation (**Fig. 1**).

It is essential for the dental practitioner to understand the etiology and management of patients with SCD. These patients are commonly misjudged when the treating health care professional does not understand SCD and how to manage patients with SCD. Dentists should collaborate with the SCD health care team to optimize the oral health care and dental experience for patients with SCD.

CLINICS CARE POINTS

- Dental treatment of patients with Sickle Cell Disease include preventive care and anxiety management.
- Severe pain is a significant symptom reported by a patient with SCD.
- Pain crisis is typically managed with parenteral opiods (morphine at 0.1 mg/kg IV or subcutaneously (SC) every 20 minutes, and maintaining this analgesia with morphine at doses of 0.05 to 0.1 mg/ kg every 2 to 4 hrs (SC/IV or PO) and nonsterioidal anti-inflammatory agents.
- Tinzaparin was found to be useful in shortening the course of pain. Oxygen saturation has to be maintained through the crisis.

DISCLOSURE

Nothing to disclose.

REFERENCES

1. Sundd P, Gladwin MT, Novelli EM. Pathophysiology of Sickle Cell Disease. Annu Rev Pathol 2019;14:263–92.

2. Kavanagh PL, Fasipe TA, Wun T. Sickle Cell Disease: A Review. JAMA 2022;328(1):57–68.
3. Piel FB, Steinberg MH, Rees DC. Sickle Cell Disease. N Engl J Med 2017;376(16):1561–73.
4. Kakkar M, Holderle K, Sheth M, et al. Orofacial Manifestation and Dental Management of Sickle Cell Disease: A Scoping Review. Anemia 2021;2021:5556708.

A Patient with Refractory Trigeminal Neuralgia was Referred for Suspected Odontogenic Pain

Stefania Brazzoli, DDS, MS[a], Lauren Levi, DMD, MS[a,*], Marlind Alan Stiles, DMD[a], Andres Pinto, DMD, MPH, MSCE, MBA[b]

KEYWORDS

- Trigeminal neuralgia • Pharmacotherapy • Refractory • Cranial nerves
- Microvascular decompression • Tooth pain

KEY POINTS

- Trigeminal neuralgia is the most common cranial nerve neuralgia.
- Patients with trigeminal neuralgia may present to a dental office complaining of dental pain.
- Patients with trigeminal neuralgia symptoms referring to tooth-bearing areas must be carefully evaluated for common dental/oral sources of pain.

CASE REPORT

A 66-year-old male presented with right-sided facial pain that started four to five years earlier. The patient believed the right facial pain started after having laser eye surgery for his right eye; he was referred initially to his general dentist, as his medical team believed the pain was odontogenic. His general dentist reported the dental evaluation was unremarkable and referred him to oral maxillofacial surgery where he was diagnosed with trigeminal neuralgia and was referred to a neurologist. The neurologist initiated him on carbamazepine and gabapentin which failed to control the patient's pain. The patient was then referred to the orofacial pain division at Thomas Jefferson University Hospital for further evaluation.

At the time of the evaluation, he described the pain as multiple episodes a day of sharp stabbing pain that lasted a few seconds separated by periods of remission.

[a] Division of Orofacial Pain, Department of Oral and Maxillofacial Pain, Thomas Jefferson University Hospital, Philadelphia, PA 19109, USA; [b] Department of Oral and Maxillofacial Medicine, Case Western Reserve University and University Hospitals Cleveland Medical Center, Cleveland, OH, USA
* Corresponding author.
E-mail address: lauren.levi@jefferson.edu

Dent Clin N Am 67 (2023) 683–685
https://doi.org/10.1016/j.cden.2023.06.004

The pain was localized to the right V1 and V2 trigeminal distributions, and the patient specifically pointed to the right nasal wall, around the right eye, right upper lip, and intraorally along the right maxilla. He reported the pain had recently worsened to more frequent attacks. He noted touching his face, brushing his teeth, chewing, eating, and stress as triggers.

The patient had tried and failed multiple medications and treatments including medical marijuana, sphenopalatine ganglion blocks, carbamazepine 400 mg three times a day, gabapentin 800 mg four times a day, and baclofen 10 mg three times a day. When he presented to the clinic, he was taking carbamazepine, baclofen, and gabapentin with poor pain control. During the general examination, the patient was well-developed, well-nourished, awake, alert, and oriented to person, place, and time. His speech was fluid and appropriate. No dysmetria on finger-to-nose testing bilaterally was noted, and he was able to stand and ambulate without assistance.

A comprehensive clinical and radiographic examination revealed no dental decay, periodontal disease, or other gross dental pathology that could account for the localized pain.

Cranial nerve screening was normal. Extraocular movements were intact without subjective diplopia or nystagmus. V1-V3 sensation was intact subjectively to light touch bilaterally. His familiar pain was reproduced upon evaluation with a refractory period noted. Muscles of facial expression were intact and symmetric bilaterally. The hearing was intact subjectively to finger rub. His tongue protruded to the midline with no deviation.

Based on his history, clinical presentation, and exclusion of other pathologies, a diagnosis of trigeminal neuralgia was confirmed.[1,2] MRI and MRA of the brain were ordered which revealed a vascular loop contacting the cisternal portion of the right fifth cranial nerve at the root entry zone. There was no evidence of mass effect or tumors.

Lamotrigine was added to his medication regimen, and the medication was titrated slowly to reduce possible adverse reactions. The patient responded positively to lamotrigine 100 twice a day. Carbamazepine was subsequently reduced, which resulted in a return of the patient's symptoms. Other medications including clonazepam and topiramate were trialed. The pharmacologic management included daily doses of carbamazepine 500 mg, lamotrigine 500 mg, gabapentin 800 mg, topiramate 50 mg, and clonazepam 0.5 mg. Despite the initial improvement in the pain with each additional medication, the patient continued to experience breakthrough pain along with cognitive side effects. The patient was referred to neurosurgery due to the refractory nature of the TN treatment and the cognitive side effects of the medications. After evaluating the case and discussing the various options for surgical intervention, including stereotactic radiosurgery, percutaneous rhizotomy, and microvascular decompression, internal neurolysis, the neurosurgeon recommended and performed microvascular decompression. At the oneweek follow-up after the MVD, the patient was asymptomatic. Patient was slowly tapered off the medications. One year follow-up post-MVD, the patient is still asymptomatic.

DENTAL MANAGEMENT DECISION AND JUSTIFICATION

The patient was managed using a multidisciplinary approach involving an orofacial pain specialist and a neurosurgeon. Initially, pharmacologic management was attempted, including prescribing carbamazepine, gabapentin, baclofen, lamotrigine, clonazepam, and topiramate. The dosage of each medication was titrated gradually to achieve pain control while monitoring systemic effects and follow-up for any adverse reactions. Additionally, the patient was advised to adopt oral hygiene practices that minimized toothbrush stimulation and to avoid triggering factors.

Despite the initial improvement in pain with each medication, the patient continued to experience breakthrough pain episodes. As a result, a referral was made to a neurosurgeon to consider surgical options such as microvascular decompression (MVD).

Trigeminal neuralgia is a debilitating pain disorder that can coexist with other oral conditions, leading to diagnostic challenges.[3] In this case, the patient's trigeminal neuralgia symptoms were initially overshadowed and misdiagnosed as possible odontogenic pain.[4] Collaboration between orofacial pain and neurosurgery was crucial to arrive at an accurate diagnosis and develop an appropriate treatment plan. Conservative medical management, including anticonvulsant medications, is often the first-line approach for TN. However, surgical interventions may be considered for refractory cases when conservative treatments fail to provide adequate pain relief or when patients cannot tolerate medications. This case highlights the successful resolution of both trigeminal neuralgia and referred tooth pain following MVD surgery, emphasizing the importance of considering multidisciplinary approaches for complex cases.

SUMMARY

Trigeminal neuralgia (TN) is a severe facial pain disorder characterized by sudden, unilateral, and electric shock-like pain in the distribution of the trigeminal nerve.[3] This case report presents a patient with typical TN symptoms, along with intraoral pain. The diagnostic process and management of the patient are discussed, emphasizing the importance of multidisciplinary collaboration for optimal patient care.

CLINICS CARE POINTS

- Trigeminal neuralgia may be present in the distribution of dental innervation. The clinician must perform a careful pain history and neurologic exam to rule out any paroxysmal component to the pain.
- A patient with suspected trigeminal neuralgia must have CNS (central nervous system) imaging to rule out a mass or vascular source for the presenting symptoms.
- A refractory period (minutes) between the activation of trigger areas is often pathognomonic for TN.

REFERENCES

1. Allam AK, Sharma H, Larkin MB, et al. Trigeminal Neuralgia: Diagnosis and Treatment. Neurol Clin 2023;41(1):107–21.
2. Araya EI, Claudino RF, Piovesan EJ, et al. Trigeminal Neuralgia: Basic and Clinical Aspects. Curr Neuropharmacol 2020;18(2):109–19.
3. Cruccu G, Di Stefano G, Truini A. Trigeminal Neuralgia. N Engl J Med 2020;383(8): 754–62.
4. Tripathi M, Sadashiva N, Gupta A, et al. Please spare my teeth! Dental procedures and trigeminal neuralgia. Surg Neurol Int 2020;11:455.

A Patient with Herpes Zoster of the Maxillary Division of Trigeminal Nerve Presents for Oral Evaluation and Toothache

Irene H. Kim, DMD, MPH[a], Archana Mupparapu, BS[b], Jana N. Yablonski, RDH[a], Mel Mupparapu, DMD, MDS, Dipl. ABOMR[a,*]

KEYWORDS

• Herpes zoster • Odontalgia • Trigeminal nerve • Odontogenic pain

KEY POINTS

- Herpes zoster (HZ) reactivated in the trigeminal nerve during the prodromal stage of the disease may mimic odontogenic pain and should be considered in the differential diagnosis.
- Thorough intraoral and extraoral examinations are essential for early diagnosis of HZ.
- Antiviral agents should be administered as early as possible to decrease the severity and duration of the HZ infection and its associated postherpetic neuralgia.
- Immunocompromised and elderly patients have a higher risk of developing HZ.

MEDICAL SCENARIO

A 55-year old man presented with intermittent throbbing pain and numbness associated with his maxillary left first molar and the left side of his face for the past 2 days. The medical history was noncontributory. Extraoral examination revealed no lymphadenopathy or neurologic deficits. Dental examination revealed fair oral hygiene with generalized plaque and conservative restorations. No intraoral lesions were noted on initial examination. Radiographic examination revealed mild to moderate generalized periodontitis, and the maxillary left posterior periapical radiograph showed no pathologic condition. Although the patient complained of paroxysms of pain in his left maxillary molar, no significant pathologic condition was noted on clinical and radiographic examination.

[a] Department of Oral Medicine, University of Pennsylvania School of Dental Medicine, Philadelphia, PA, USA; [b] Temple University School of Medicine, Philadelphia, PA, USA
* Corresponding author. Department of Oral Medicine, Penn Dental Medicine, 240 South 40th Street, Philadelphia, PA 19104.
E-mail address: mmd@upenn.edu

Dent Clin N Am 67 (2023) 687–690
https://doi.org/10.1016/j.cden.2023.05.022
dental.theclinics.com

DENTAL MANAGEMENT DECISION AND JUSTIFICATION

The patient was referred to the Department of Oral Medicine for evaluation of possible trigeminal neuralgia. At his appointment the following day, the patient presented with extraoral lesions on the left side of his face and intraoral lesions isolated to the left side of his hard palate following the dermatome of the left maxillary division of the trigeminal nerve. This led to a preliminary diagnosis of Herpes Zoster (HZ), which was later confirmed with laboratory testing, and the patient was treated with famciclovir.

HZ, commonly known as shingles, is a reactivation of the latent Varicella-zoster virus (VZV), which is spread via respiratory droplets and often manifests as varicella, or chickenpox. VZV remains dormant and asymptomatic in dorsal root or cranial nerve ganglia until it reactivates in patients who are often immunocompromised or elderly.[1] Clinical symptoms of HZ begin during a prodromal stage, which may present as itching, burning, or pain at the affected dermatome. Additional symptoms may include headaches, general malaise, and photophobia.[2] In the following days or weeks, the patient develops painful vesicles in a unilateral, bandlike pattern across the dermatome.[1] This acute phase may continue for several weeks, and if severe pain remains for longer than 4 weeks, the infection enters the chronic stage. With chronic HZ or postherpetic neuralgia (PNH), the patient may experience dysesthesias, paresthesias, and shocklike sensations in addition to the severe pain.[2]

Laboratory testing options for HZ (**Box 1**) include polymerase chain reaction (PCR), direct fluorescent antigen (DFA), and viral culture. PCR testing is the preferred choice owing to its high sensitivity and specificity, availability, and turnaround times averaging less than 1 day.[1,2] DFA testing is a less-sensitive alternative to PCR testing, but is still acceptable if PCR is not available. Viral culture testing is the least preferred option because of its low sensitivity and the longest turnaround time, with cultures taking 3 to 14 days for growth.

Box 1
Summary of herpes zoster presenting as a toothache, the testing and treatment of HZ in order of preference, and the vaccinations that are currently available

HZ of maxillary branch of trigeminal nerve mimicking a toothache
- Prodromal stage: Toothache and facial pain with no lesions.
  Duration 1 to 2 days
- Acute stage: Painful eruption of vesicles extraorally/intraorally following the dermatome of the maxillary branch of the nerve.
  Duration 2 to 4 weeks
- Chronic stage: Severe and often debilitating pain, known as post-herpetic neuralgia (PHN)
  Duration >4 weeks, often lasting months

Testing in order of preference
- PCR: Highest sensitivity and specificity with <1-day turnaround
- DFA: Suitable alternative to PCR, better sensitivity than viral culture with shorter turnaround
- Viral culture: Least sensitive, difficult to collect specimen, long turnaround of 3 to 14 days

Treatment in order of preference
- Oral famciclovir: 500 mg 3 times daily for 1 week
  Or
  Oral valacyclovir: 1 g 3 times daily for 1 week
- Oral acyclovir: 800 mg 5 times daily for 1 week

Vaccination: 2 types available
- Zostavaz, live-attenuated VZV vaccine
- Shingrix, recombinant adjuvanted VZV vaccine
- Recommended for adults aged 50 years or older

HZ vaccines are available for the prevention of HZ and are strongly recommended (see **Box 1**). Treatment of HZ is with oral antiviral agents, preferably within 72 hours of lesion onset. Famciclovir and valacyclovir are preferred owing to their simpler dosing schedules (see **Box 1**) and better pharmacokinetic characteristics, but acyclovir is a suitable substitute if neither famciclovir nor valacyclovir is available.[1,2] Topical antiviral therapy has been found to be ineffective and is not recommended. Intravenous antivirals should be given only to immunocompromised patients with severe HZ presentation, and/or HZ complicated by central nervous system involvement.[1] Neuralgic pain can be acute, and acetaminophen or ibuprofen can be taken for pain management.

Most HZ infections occur in the thoracic and lumbar dermatomes, but about 13% occur in the branches of the trigeminal nerve.[3] The ophthalmic branch is most commonly affected, but in some cases, the maxillary branch is involved. During the prodromal period before the outbreak of mucocutaneous lesions, the patient can experience sensations such as burning, itching, or numbness along the cutaneous distribution of the dermatome. If the maxillary branch of the trigeminal nerve is affected during this prodromal stage, odontalgia and pulpal necrosis may occur. This presents a diagnostic challenge for dentists.

It is very difficult to diagnose HZ during the prodromal stage when a dental patient may complain of tooth pain,[4] but HZ should be included in the differential diagnosis particularly if the patient is immunocompromised or elderly. Early detection and treatment of HZ decreases the severity and duration of an HZ infection and its associated post-herpetic neuralgia (PHN).[5] In the above medical scenario, a conservative dental approach was taken in the absence of clinical or radiographic evidence of an obvious infection. The outbreak of unilateral lesions the following day led to the diagnosis of HZ. The lesions and odontogenic pain resolved with antiviral therapy within 3 weeks, but the patient developed postherpetic neuralgia, which was managed with analgesics. In the absence of an obvious odontogenic infection in patients presenting with odontalgia, dentists should consider the possibility of HZ involving the maxillary branch of the trigeminal nerve.

CLINICS CARE POINTS

- Herpes Zoster, commonly known as Shingles is a reactivation of the latent Varicella-Zoster Virus (VZC) that spreads via respiratory droplets. The condition can be prevented via vaccination and highly recommended for patients 50 yrs or older.
- There are two available vaccines for preventiona. Live attenuated VZC vaccine andb. Recombinant adjuvanted VZC vaccine.Both are equally efficacious.
- Oral femciclovir 500 mg t.i.d for one week is the treatment of choice. Oral acyclovir is an alternate drug of choice with doses ranging from 800mg taken 5 times daily for one week or 1 gram t.i.d. for one week.
- Post-Herpetic Neuralgia (PHN) is a common complication of Herpes Zoster.

DISCLOSURE

The authors have nothing to disclose.

REFERENCES

1. Schmader K. Herpes Zoster. Ann Intern Med 2018;169(3):516–33.
2. Patil A, Goldust M, Wollina U. Herpes Zoster: A Review of Clinical Manifestations and Management. Viruses 2022;14(2):192–205.

3. Millar EP, Troulis MJ. Herpes zoster of the trigeminal nerve: the dentist's role in diagnosis and treatment. J Can Dent Assoc 1994;60(5):450–3.
4. Fristad I, Bardsen A, Knudsen GC, et al. Prodromal herpes zoster - a diagnostic challenge in endodontics. Int Endod J 2002;12:1012–7.
5. Mustafa MB, Arduino PG, Porter SR. Varicella zoster virus: review of its management. J Oral Pathol Med 2009;38(9):673–88.

Child Patient with a History of Status Epilepticus Referred for Management of Grossly Decayed Primary Molar

Elizabeth Bortell, DDS[a,*],
Jayakumar Jayaraman, BDS, MDS, FDSRCS, MS, PhD[a]

KEYWORDS

- Status epilepticus • Seizures • General anesthesia • Epilepsy • Children • Dental

KEY POINTS

- Patients with status epilepticus are at risk for sustained seizure activity that can be life threatening.
- Physician consultation is needed before treatment of a patient with status epilepticus.
- General anesthesia should be considered if seizures are uncontrolled and treatment needs are extensive.

MEDICAL SCENARIO

A 5-year-old boy presents for an initial examination.

Chief Complaint

"My tooth hurts."

The patient indicated his upper right primary second molar by pointing. The mother stated that the pain occurs while eating and is alleviated with over-the-counter nonsteroidal anti-inflammatory drugs. The mother denies any history of unprovoked spontaneous or nocturnal pain. Patient had a history of a dental visit several years ago. Mother stated that the visit did not go well, and she did not return for dental care. Mother reports that the patient has seizures that last for several minutes and has them often. She indicated that she did not know the type of seizures and provided very little historical information. History of one hospitalization for uncontrolled seizures was reported by the mother.

[a] Department of Pediatric Dentistry, Virginia Commonwealth University, 1101 E Leigh Street, Richmond, VA 23298-0566, USA
* Corresponding author. Department of Pediatric Dentistry, Virginia Commonwealth University School of Dentistry, 1101 E Leigh Street, Richmond, VA 23298-0566.
E-mail address: ebbortell@vcu.edu

Dent Clin N Am 67 (2023) 691–694
https://doi.org/10.1016/j.cden.2023.05.024
dental.theclinics.com

Patient had no known drug allergies. Patient was prescribed valproic acid (Depakote); diazepam (Diastat) in prior visits. Extraoral examination was unremarkable. No facial swelling or lymphadenopathy. Intraoral examination showed primary dentition, mesial step occlusion, gross caries on maxillary right primary second molar, occlusal caries in other primary molars. Possible other carious teeth pending radiographic examination.

Bitewing radiographs were not obtained in the dental setting due to poor patient behavior. Able to acquire a bitewing radiograph in the operating room under general anesthesia that revealed caries of the maxillary right primary second molar, tooth #A involving the distal pulp horn. Caries also noted involving enamel and dentin in the mesial surfaces of tooth #B, #S, and #T. No furcal or periapical radiolucency noted in any of the teeth (**Fig. 1**).

Diagnosis

Dental caries in tooth #B, #S, and #T. Dental caries in tooth #A with reversible pulpitis.

Behavior

Frankl Behavior Rating Scale 2 (Negative).[1] Reluctance to accept treatment, uncooperative, showing some negativity.

Dental management decision and justification.

Tentative Treatment Plan

Obtain consultation from Neurologist regarding patient's seizure type, frequency, seizure history, medications, seizure triggers, and recommendation for management with local anesthesia and possible general anesthesia.

Medical Consultation

Medical consultation was obtained from the patient's neurologist indicating the patient's diagnosis of status epilepticus. History of hospitalization 1 year ago due to uncontrolled and prolonged seizures. Patient has recurrent refractory seizures that are regularly that are not provoked by any stimuli. The seizures are currently managed with valproic acid and Diastat as needed for seizures lasting longer than 5 minutes.

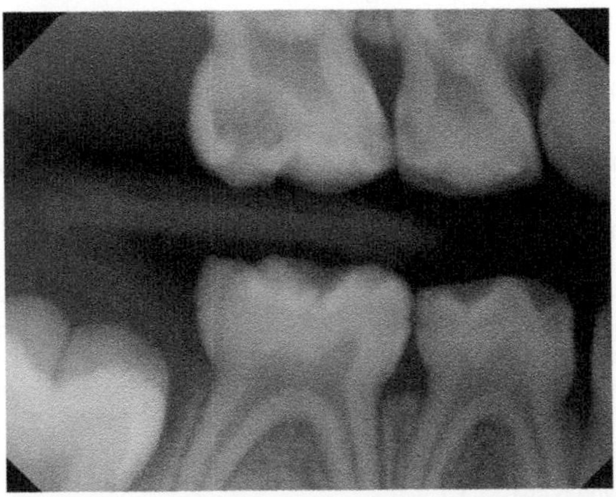

Fig. 1. Bitewing radiograph showing caries in distal of tooth #A involving the distal pulp horn, mesial caries in #B, #S, and #T.

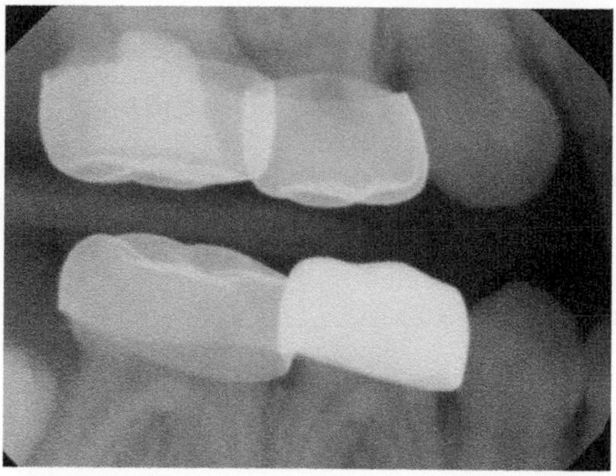

Fig. 2. Bitewing radiograph showing formocresol pulpotomy in tooth #A with stainless steel crown, and stainless-steel crowns in #B, #S, and #T.

The neurologist recommended treatment under general anesthesia in a hospital setting if the patient requires admission for seizure management after treatment. The neurologist also cautioned the use of lidocaine, which lowers the seizure threshold, and recommended laboratories to evaluate platelet count because valproic acid can decrease the platelet count.

Comprehensive Treatment Plan

The patient was scheduled in an acute care hospital that would allow for hospitalization if needed. Platelet counts were in normal range and the patient was cleared for the procedure by the history and physical. Treatment under general anesthesia included clinical and radiographic examination, prophylaxis, and fluoride application. Rubber dam was placed, caries was excavated in tooth #A, and coronal pulp was approached and removed. Hemostasis was achieved with sterile wet cotton pellet, and diluted Formocresol (48.5% Formaldehyde, 48.5% cresol, 3% Glycerine) was placed for 5 minutes. Following this, intermediate restorative material was placed, and stainless-steel crowns was cemented on maxillary right primary second molar, tooth #A. Stainless steel crowns were also placed on the maxillary right primary first molar, mandibular right primary first and second molar (**Fig. 2**). On completion of treatment, the patient was discharged without need for admission.

DISCUSSION

Patients with status epilepticus are at risk for life threatening and prolonged seizure activity.[2] Lidocaine may lower the seizure threshold if given in toxic levels or intravascularly.[3] There is also a risk of low platelet counts and bleeding complications for those patients taking valproic acid.[2] Patients with status epilepticus have an American Society of Anesthesiologist classification of III or IV, and therefore, treatment under general anesthesia with possible admission should be considered[3]; particularly if the patient has multiple carious lesions, and if age and behavior limit routine care. Moreover, the most definitive treatment should be planned to prevent future need for retreatment due to treatment failure or recurrent caries. Medical consultation should always be obtained for any patient with seizure disorder to obtain information about the type, frequency, history, including the last seizure, medications, and any known precipitating factors.[2]

REFERENCES

1. Wright G, Stingers J. Nonpharmacologic management of children's behaviors. In: Dean J, Avery D, McDonal R, editors. McDonald and avery's dentistry for the child and adolescent. Missouri: Mosby; 2011. p. 28.
2. Moursi AM. Clinical cases in pediatric dentistry. In: da Fonseca MA, Truesdale AL, editors. Seizure disorder, intellectual disability. United Kingdom: Blackwell Publishing; 2012. p. 285–9.
3. Kennedy B, Haller J. Treatment of the epileptic patient in the dental office. N Y State Dent J 1998;64(2):26–31.

Patient with Crohn's Disease Presents for Pain in Relation to Maxillary Teeth

Payam Mirfendereski, DDS[a], Lauren Wilson, MSN, CRNP[b], Katherine France, DMD, MBE[a,*]

KEYWORDS

- Inflammatory bowel disease • Oral manifestations • Orofacial granulomatosis
- Oral health–related quality of life • Referred pain • Crohn's disease

KEY POINTS

- Crohn's disease is a chronic inflammatory bowel condition that may present with oral lesions.
- Classic oral lesions associated with Crohn's disease include mucosal tags, mucosal cobblestoning, mucogingivitis, linear ulcerations, and cheilitis granulomatosa.
- Nonspecific oral lesions associated with Crohn's disease include aphthous ulcers, angular cheilitis, and pyostomatitis vegetans.
- Some of the oral manifestations of Crohn's disease tend to be asymptomatic, whereas mucosal ulcerations and orofacial granulomatosis can be painful and have a significant impact on patients' quality of life.

MEDICAL SCENARIO

A 28-year-old woman arrives to the dental clinic complaining of chronic and worsening pain in her upper front teeth, pointing to #10 and #11. She describes the pain as a sharp, 7/10 pain, aggravated by eating and drinking that has been present for approximately 8 months. She has not noticed any intraoral swelling or bleeding, but reports that she woke up with a particularly swollen upper lip today (**Fig. 1**), and she endorses waxing and waning upper lip swelling over the past year. She reports intermittent ulcers on her labial and buccal mucosa. Her medical history is significant only for Crohn's disease, currently managed by her gastroenterologist with infliximab infusions every 8 weeks for the last 3 years without recent symptom flares. She reports that she

[a] Department of Oral Medicine, University of Pennsylvania School of Dental Medicine, 240 South 40th Street, Philadelphia, PA 19104, USA; [b] Division of Gastroenterology, Hospital of the University of Pennsylvania, Center for Inflammatory Bowel Disease, 3400 Spruce Street, Philadelphia, PA 19104, USA
* Corresponding author.
E-mail address: kfrance@upenn.edu

Dent Clin N Am 67 (2023) 695–698
https://doi.org/10.1016/j.cden.2023.05.026

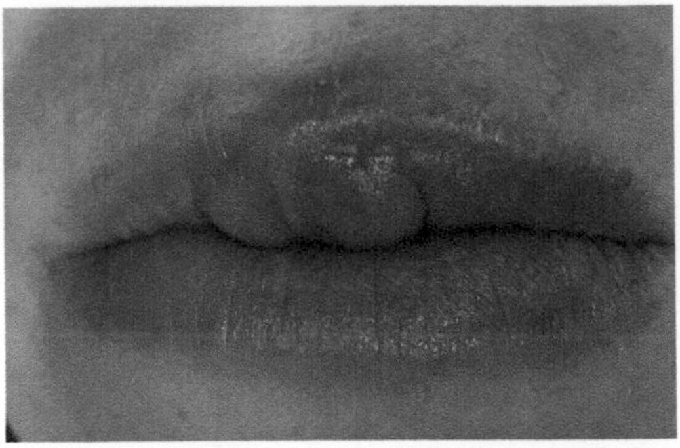

Fig. 1. Extraoral lip swelling, particularly notable on the upper lip, in a patient with orofacial granulomatosis as can be associated with Crohn's disease.

often finds it difficult to eat a proper meal due to her oral pain, causing her to lose 20 pounds in the last 6 months. She denies any other recent systemic symptoms or changes.

DENTAL MANAGEMENT DECISION AND JUSTIFICATION

A comprehensive dental evaluation must be performed to evaluate this patient's complaints and rule out any odontogenic cause. In order to appropriately complete this evaluation, the dentist must be familiar with the possibility of referred nonodontogenic pain in a patient with Crohn's disease. Crohn's disease is a chronic inflammatory bowel condition that can affect any aspect of the gastrointestinal tract, with lesions most common in the distal ileum and colon.[1] Multifactorial in cause, Crohn's disease has been linked to various genetic, environmental, bacterial, and immunological factors.[2] It can be a debilitating condition, and although gastrointestinal symptoms such as diarrhea and abdominal pain predominate, other organ systems ranging from the eyes to the skin and joints as well as others can also be implicated in approximately one-quarter of affected patients.[3]

Oral lesions classically associated with Crohn's disease include mucosal tags, mucosal cobblestoning, mucogingivitis, linear ulcerations, and cheilitis granulomatosa. Certain nonspecific oral lesions such as aphthous ulcers, angular cheilitis, and pyostomatitis vegetans can also be seen in patients with Crohn's disease.[4] Mucogingivitis can present as hyperplastic and granular gingiva extending from the gingival margin to the mucogingival junction. The linear ulcerations present in Crohn's disease are most commonly seen in the buccal and labial vestibules.[4] Cheilitis granulomatosa presents as lip swelling and is a subset of orofacial granulomatosis, a condition involving noncaseating granulomatous inflammation.[5] Orofacial granulomatosis can be varyingly disfiguring and painful, at times severely affecting the patient's quality of life. Both the upper and lower lips can be affected, although the lower lip has a slightly higher incidence.[5] The lip swelling is initially recurrent and edematous but becomes persistent and granular over time. Along with the labial swelling, perpendicular ulcerations can occur on the lip in orofacial granulomatosis. Although some of the orofacial manifestations of Crohn's disease are associated with minimal symptoms, both mucosal ulcerations and orofacial granulomatosis can be possible causes for the above patient's complaint of pain associated with her anterior maxillary teeth.

The goal of Crohn's disease treatment is to control inflammation and alter disease progression early in order to minimize complications including stricturing, fistulization, neoplasia, and need for surgery. Biological therapies are effective at inducing and maintaining remission; commonly used medications include infliximab, adalimumab, and certolizumab (anti-tumor necrosis factor-α therapy), ustekinumab (anti–IL-12/-23 monoclonal therapy), vedolizumab (gut-specific anti--ntegrin $\alpha 4\beta 7$ monoclonal therapy) and risankizumab (anti–IL-23 monoclonal therapy). Immunomodulators such as methotrexate and thiopurines, when used as monotherapy, are less effective than biologics. Mesalamine therapy has been shown to be an ineffective treatment option.[6] Surgical interventions such as stricturoplasty or resection of affected areas may also be considered, especially in refractory or fibrotic stricturing disease. For the oral manifestations of Crohn's disease, topical or intralesional corticosteroids or other topical immunosuppressants are frequently used as adjuncts to systemic therapy. Surgical cheiloplasty and low-level laser therapy are also possible treatment options for orofacial granulomatosis.[5] It is important to note that oral manifestations of Crohn's disease do not necessarily correlate with the level of gastrointestinal disease activity, and patients may develop active oral disease even when gastrointestinal symptoms are well controlled.[4]

Crohn's disease has been associated with poor oral health and oral health–related quality of life.[7] Although the specific and nonspecific oral manifestations of Crohn's disease can be sources of referred pain, patients with Crohn's disease also tend to have higher rates of periodontitis and caries and have been found to exhibit increased salivary composition of *Streptococcus mutans* and *Lactobacillus* species, which may result from either changes in diet or reduced microbial diversity and increased dysbiosis.[8] Crohn's disease has been associated with an increased risk for initiation and progression of periodontal disease due to certain genetic and environmental factors, microbial dysbiosis, and overactive host response.[2] The higher prevalence of caries has been attributed to nutritional and behavioral predilections as well as associated salivary and microbiological alterations.[2] Working with this patient to modify caries and periodontal risk factors and educating her on the orofacial manifestations of Crohn's disease could be especially beneficial in improving her oral health–related quality of life.

CLINICS CARE POINTS

- Crohn's disease is an inflammatory bowel condition that can present with a variety of oral manifestations.
- Management of oral lesions in Crohn's disease may be required together with or separate from systemic management.
- Oral and periodontal health can be compromised in Crohn's disease and must be carefully monitored.

CONFLICT OF INTEREST

All authors declare that they have no commercial or financial conflict of interest related to the material in this article and have received no funding for the preparation of this article.

REFERENCES

1. Jajam M, Bozzolo P, Niklander S. Oral Manifestations of Gastrointestinal Disorders. J Clin Exp Dent 2017;9(10):e1242–8.

2. Papageorgiou SN, Hagner M, Nogueira AV, et al. Inflammatory bowel disease and oral health: systematic review and a meta-analysis. J Clin Periodontol 2017;44(4): 382–93.
3. Rogler G, Singh A, Kavanaugh A, et al. Extraintestinal Manifestations of Inflammatory Bowel Disease: Current Concepts, Treatment, and Implications for Disease Management. Gastroenterology 2021;161(4):1118–32.
4. Lauritano D, Boccalari E, Di Stasio D, et al. Prevalence of Oral Lesions and Correlation with Intestinal Symptoms of Inflammatory Bowel Disease: A Systematic Review. Diagnostics 2019;9(3):77.
5. Al-Hamad A, Porter S, Fedele S. Orofacial Granulomatosis. Dermatol Clin 2015; 33(3):433–46.
6. Cushing K, Higgins PDR. Management of Crohn Disease: A Review. JAMA 2021; 325(1):69–80.
7. Nijakowski K, Gruszczyński D, Surdacka A. Oral Health Status in Patients with Inflammatory Bowel Diseases: A Systematic Review. Int J Environ Res Public Health 2021;18(21):11521.
8. Marruganti C, Discepoli N, Gaeta C, et al. Dental Caries Occurrence in Inflammatory Bowel Disease Patients: A Systematic Review and Meta-Analysis. Caries Res 2021;55(5):485–95.

A Patient Diagnosed with Bulimia Reports to the Dental Office Seeking Cosmetic Dental Work

Irene H. Kim, DMD, MPH[a], Walter W. Hong, MD, Dipl. ABPN[b], Mel Mupparapu, DMD, MDS, Dipl. ABOMR[a,*]

KEYWORDS

• Bulimia • Eating disorders • Dental erosion • Perimylolysis • Sialadenosis

KEY POINTS

- Bulimia nervosa (BN) is a serious psychiatric illness that is 1 of 8 eating disorders recognized by the Diagnostic and Statistical Manual of Mental Disorders 5th edition.
- The self-induced vomiting in BN and its associated binge eating result in dental manifestations of the disease that dentists should recognize.
- Common oral manifestations include dental erosion, dental caries, parotid gland hypertrophy, and trauma to the oral mucosa.
- Treatment of BN is multidisciplinary to treat the medical and dental complications and includes psychopharmacologic and psychotherapeutic treatments of the BN behavior.

MEDICAL SCENARIO

An anxious 23-year-old woman presented to the clinic with a chief complaint of "sensitive teeth" and "wanting to fix her teeth." Her past medical history was significant for a diagnosis of bulimia nervosa (BN) 5 years ago when she was a student athlete. She stated that her BN is now being managed with her psychiatrist and family doctor. She is currently taking fluoxetine and has no known drug allergies. Intraoral examination revealed mildly erythematous mucosa, gingivitis, palatal erosion on the anterior maxillary dentition with chipping of the incisal edges, and mild occlusal erosion of the maxillary posterior dentition. On extraoral examination, the parotid gland seemed enlarged, slight redness in her eyes was detected, and a callous was observed on a knuckle of her right hand. As she related her history of BN and discussed treatment options, she seemed to become more relaxed and less anxious.

[a] Department of Oral Medicine, University of Pennsylvania School of Dental Medicine, Penn Dental Medicine, 240 South 40th Street, Philadelphia, PA 19104, USA; [b] Replimune, Clinical Development, Woburn, MA, USA
* Corresponding author.
E-mail address: mmd@upenn.edu

Dent Clin N Am 67 (2023) 699–702
https://doi.org/10.1016/j.cden.2023.05.027

Abbreviations	
BN	Bulimia nervosa
ED	Eating disorder
DSM	Diagnostic and statistical manual of mental disorders

DENTAL MANAGEMENT DECISION AND JUSTIFICATION

The patient was treated with conservative anterior composite restorations to improve the sensitivity from the perimylolysis or dental erosion and referred to the Department of Restorative Dentistry for treatment planning of possible veneers or crowns. Routine dental visits were strongly encouraged, and oral hygiene instructions were reinforced due to the xerostomia that may be caused by her medication. Custom fluoride trays were also delivered to help prevent future caries. The patient was encouraged to maintain a good relationship with the clinic to help her reach her goals of managing her BN and ultimately restoring her smile with veneers and crowns.

BN is a serious mental health disorder that is among 8 eating disorders (EDs) recognized by the Diagnostic and Statistical Manual of Mental Disorders 5th edition (DSM-5). Patients with BN will repeatedly (at least once a week for 3 months according to the DSM-5) eat an objectively large amount of food and then take inappropriate compensatory steps to prevent weight gain, such as vomiting, fasting, or excessive exercising.[1] During these episodes, patients with BN feel that they are not in control of their bingeing and purging. This behavior often occurs in secret, and patients often feel ashamed or disgusted after a binge and purge. The severity of BN is graded based on number of vomiting episodes per week (**Box 1**).[2] BN and ED usually develop in adolescence and early adulthood with an approximate female

Box 1
Summary of the signs, grades of severity, systemic, and dental effects of bulimia nervosa

Signs of BN
- Russell sign—callous on dorsal aspect of fingers from repeated attempts to induce vomiting
- "Chipmunk-type" face—from sialadenosis, parotid gland swelling
- Subconjunctival hemorrhage and epistaxis from frequent vomiting strain

Grading of severity purging episodes per week
- Mild 1 to 3
- Moderate 4 to 7
- Severe 8 to 13
- Extreme 14 or more

Systemic effects
- Electrolyte imbalances—metabolic alkalosis, hypokalemia
- Gastric and esophageal rupture
- Dizziness, excessive thirst, syncope
- Colitis, pancreatitis
- Cardiovascular and renal failure in severe cases

Dental effects
- Perimylolysis, dental erosion of tooth surfaces
- Hypersensitivity of teeth
- Dental caries
- Sialadenosis, parotid gland hypertrophy
- Xerostomia

to male ratio of 10:1.[2] The prevalence of BN has been reported to be 1% to 1.5% in adults and 1% to 2% in adolescents, but other studies on ED that do not use the DSM-5 have reported a prevalence of 14% to 22%.[1] Among the comorbidities associated with BN in adolescents, mood and anxiety disorders were the highest, with 53% reporting suicidal ideation.[1]

The systemic effects of BN, which stem primarily from the purging behavior, can be observed on physical examination and in laboratory test results[2] (see **Box 1**). The self-induced vomiting also will cause esophagitis, esophageal erosions, and bleeding. In severe cases, cardiovascular and renal failure may occur.[2]

Oral manifestations of BN also stem primarily from the self-induced vomiting behavior, which include perimylolysis, dental hypersensitivity, dental caries, sialadenosis, xerostomia, and periodontitis.[2,3] Perimylolysis, or dental erosion, is a common oral finding because the gastric acid that is purged into the oral cavity has a pH of 2.9, which is far less than the critical pH of 5.5 necessary to dissolve dental enamel. The teeth most affected by perimylolysis are the maxillary teeth with the palatal surfaces of the maxillary anterior dentition most severely affected. The mandibular dentition may be affected, but it is often protected by the tongue during the purging episodes. Patients with BN may also experience a higher caries rate due to the high carbohydrate consumption during a binge, poor oral hygiene, and the xerostomia that can occur from their medication.

The treatment of BN is multidisciplinary, which includes psychosocial and psychopharmacologic approaches.[4] Psychosocial treatments can include cognitive behavioral therapy, group psychotherapy, family therapy, and support groups. The medications often prescribed are antidepressants such as tricyclic antidepressants, selective serotonin reuptake inhibitors, and monoamine oxidase inhibitors. Nutritionists and dieticians are involved to help educate patients with BN on proper eating habits. These patients also should be seen by medical professionals to address the systemic manifestations of their behavior such as electrolyte imbalances, esophageal issues, and in severe cases cardiovascular and renal failure.

Dental professionals should be aware of the oral manifestations secondary to the purging behavior and xerostomia from the medications, including careful monitoring of the perimylolysis as well as dental caries. Dentists are also in a unique position not only to recognize signs of ED and BN but also to support and encourage their patients. There is a general stigma toward mental disorders, and in ED and BN this has a harmful impact on the patients' self-esteem and treatment seeking behavior.[5] Dentists should be knowledgeable about EDs and BN to help improve the diagnosis and treatment of their patents with such a condition.

CLINICS CARE POINTS

- Bulimia and other eating disorders are psychiatric illnessess manifested by disordered and disturbed attitides of eating and body image usually accompanied by extreme methods of weight control.
- Patients with eating disorders are considered medically compromised due to the risk of grave medical complications related to cardiac arrhythmias or cardiac arrest secondary to electrolyte imbalance.
- In-office Fluoride varnish applications, home application of neutral fluoride and use of calcium phosphate products to promote remineralization and relieve dental hypersensitivity are recommended in addition to salivary stimulants for treatment of xerostomia.

DISCLOSURE

Nothing to disclose.

REFERENCES

1. Hail L, Le Grange D. Bulimia nervosa in adolescents: prevalence and treatment challenges. Adolesc Health Med Ther 2018;9:11–6.
2. Ranalli DN, Studen-Pavlovich D. Eating disorders in the adolescent patient. Dent Clin North Am 2021;65(4):689–703.
3. Rosten A, Newton T. The impact of bulimia nervosa on oral health: A review of the literature. Br Dent J 2017;223(7):533–9.
4. Yager J, Devlin MJ, Halmi KA, et al. Practice guideline for the treatment of patients with eating disorders. Am J Psychiatry. 2006;163(7 Suppl):4-54.
5. Brelet L, Flaudias V, Désert M, et al. Stigmatization toward people with anorexia nervosa, bulimia nervosa, and binge eating disorder: a scoping review. Nutrients 2021;13(8):2834.

A Pregnant Patient (First Trimester) Reporting for Pain in Relation to the Maxillary Left First Molar Was Prescribed a Full Mouth Series Radiographs in the Dental Office

Peter W. Duda, DMD[a], Steven R. Singer, DDS[a],
Eman Alamodi, BDS[b], Mel Mupparapu, DMD, MDS, Dipl. ABOMR[b,*]

KEYWORDS

• Dental radiographs • Radiographic selection criteria • Radiographs and pregnancy • Radiation safety • Radiation dose • Dental considerations in pregnancy • ALADA-IP

KEY POINTS

- Patient management during pregnancy; prudent selection and prescription of radiographic imaging to arrive at a definitive diagnosis regarding the chief complaint; presentation of viable treatment options with accompanying risks and benefits.

MEDICAL SCENARIO

A 32-year-old female patient presented with a complaint of pain of several days' duration in her upper left posterior tooth. The patient reports lingering pain to chewing and thermal fluctuation. The symptoms were alleviated by over-the-counter analgesics. Medical history revealed that the patient is approximately 2 months pregnant, after in vitro fertilization. In addition, the patient has suffered 2 prior miscarriages and is apprehensive in consenting to dental radiographs.

DENTAL MANAGEMENT DECISION AND JUSTIFICATION

On presenting to a dental office, the patient was informed that, per the rules of the office, all new patients must have a full mouth series of intraoral radiographs taken

[a] Rutgers University School of Dental Medicine; [b] Department of Oral Medicine, Penn Dental Medicine, 240 South 40th Street, Philadelphia, PA 19104, USA
* Corresponding author.
E-mail address: mmd@upenn.edu

Dent Clin N Am 67 (2023) 703–705
https://doi.org/10.1016/j.cden.2023.05.028

before being seen by the dentist. The patient expressed reluctance to receiving the radiographs. Acknowledging the patient's concerns regarding dental radiographs, she was informed by the office manager that the radiation dose would be very minimal. The patient reluctantly acquiesced to the radiographs, and the images were exposed by a licensed dental assistant. Although a digital image receptor and a lead apron and thyroid collar were used for the examination, there was no rectangular collimator in place. Round collimation imparts approximately 3 times the dose of ionizing radiation compared with a rectangular collimation.[1] The dentist introduced herself and performed an extraoral and intraoral examination. Based on the radiographic appearance of the fractured multisurface restoration with recurrent caries, and positive responses to pulp tests, the maxillary left first molar was determined to be the source of the patient's pain. The patient was afebrile with negative lymphadenopathy. Based on the radiographic and clinical data, a definitive diagnosis of symptomatic irreversible pulpitis and symptomatic apical periodontitis was confirmed.

The clinical and radiographic examination revealed that the patient had multiple carious lesions with generalized moderate to heavy plaque and calculus accumulation. The gingival tissues were erythematous with blunted papillae and bled easily on manipulation. The patient was presented with viable treatment options of either endodontic treatment and subsequent restoration of the tooth or extraction. All accompanying risks and benefits of the proposed treatment options were explained. The patient consented to endodontic therapy on the maxillary left first molar. Under local anesthesia and rubber dam isolation, the canals were identified, debrided, and irrigated with sodium hypochlorite, filled with calcium hydroxide, sealed with a protective restoration with occlusal adjustment. The patient was given oral hygiene and plaque control instructions. All elective dental therapies were postponed until after delivery.

IDEAL MANAGEMENT

Pregnancy creates an assortment of physiologic and oral changes in the dental patient. Clinicians need to have a good understanding of the physiologic changes in the body, as well as the effects of ionizing radiation and prescribed medications. The potential for radiation effects exist although the risk from dental imaging can be considered very minimal when proper radiation protection protocols are followed. These include thyroid and abdominal shielding, use of fast image receptors (photostimulable phosphors [PSP], charge coupled devices [CCD], or complementary metaloxide semiconductors [CMOS] digital sensors), rectangular collimation, use of aligning instruments, and proper radiographic selection criteria.[2] Because of the potential for radiation exposure to the pregnant patient, dental imaging should be limited to diagnosis and treatment planning of only emergent conditions.[3–5] Clinicians should conduct a detailed history and clinical examination that will direct the appropriate and selective radiographic imaging required.[6] In this case scenario, the dentist did not prescribe radiographs considering the emergent situation only. Elective radiographs were also taken. Furthermore, the risk from ionizing radiation can be minimized with the abovementioned radiation safety protocols (lead shielding, thyroid collar and rectangular collimation, in addition to the use of aligning instruments), as well as adhering to both the ALARA (As Low As Reasonably Achievable) and ALADA (As Low As Diagnostically Acceptable) principles. Once urgent conditions have been palliated, definitive dental treatment can likely be deferred until after delivery.

CLINICS CARE POINTS

- Selective radiography should be followed in dental practice rather than routine radiography. FDA/ADA guidelines must be followed when prescribing dental radiographs.
- Pregnancy brings in significant physiologic and oral changes in the dental patient. All emergent radiogaphs should be taken that will aid in diagnosis and dental treatment planning for the pregnant patient. All elective dental treatment can likely be deferred.
- Thyroid and abdominal shielding, use of fast digital image receptors, rectangular collimation, use of aligning instruments are recommended apart from following proper radiographic selection criteria.

DISCLOSURE

None.

REFERENCES

1. Magill D, Ngo NJH, Felice MA, et al. Kerma area product (KAP) and scatter measurements for intraoral X-ray machines using three different types of round collimation compared with rectangular beam limiter. Dentomaxillofac Radiol 2019;48(2): 20180183.
2. American Dental Association Council on Scientific Affairs. The use of dental radiographs: update and recommendations. J Am Dent Assoc 2006;137(9):1304–12.
3. Bahanan L, Tehsin A, Mousa R, et al. Women's awareness regarding the use of dental imaging during pregnancy. BMC Oral Health 2021;21(1):357.
4. Hemalatha VT. Dental considerations in pregnancy-a critical review on the oral care. J Clin Diagn Res 2013;7(5):948–53.
5. Serman NJ, Singer S. Exposure of the pregnant patient to ionizing radiation. Ann Dent 1994;53(2):13–5.
6. Kim IH, Mupparapu M. Dental radiographic guidelines: a review. Quintessence Int 2009;40(5):389–98.

[illegible]

A Pregnant Patient with Gestational Diabetes Reports for Scaling and Root Planning

Milda Chmieliauskaite, DMD, MPH[a,*],
Marie D. Grosh, DNP, APRN-CNP, LNHA[b], Ali Syed, BDS, MHA, MS[c],
Andres Pinto, DMD, MPH, MSCE, MBA[c]

KEYWORDS

- Gestational diabetes • Periodontal disease • Periodontal treatment

KEY POINTS

- Individuals with gestational diabetes are encouraged to receive oral health care to control oral disease during pregnancy.
- Assessment of blood sugar control in gestational diabetes differs from assessment in established adults with diabetes mellitus.
- Dentists can gauge the level of glycemic control by assessing what the blood sugar levels have been over the last 2 weeks.

MEDICAL SCENARIO

A 34-year-old female patient presents to her dentist for select scaling and root planning to treat stage I periodontal disease. She has not had a dental visit in the last 2 years. Her medical history is positive for multigravida (second pregnancy at 28 weeks gestation) and gestational diabetes mellitus. Medications include prenatal vitamins. Family history is positive for diabetes mellitus type II on her maternal side. Her vitals were stable, and she reports that her blood sugar ranged between 120 and 140 mg/dL 1 hour postprandial during the last week. On physical examination findings included 5 mm periodontal probing depths with select areas of bleeding on probing around the posterior molars.

[a] University of Washington Department of Oral Medicine School of Dentistry, Box 356370, 1959 NE Pacific Street, Seattle, WA 98195-6370, USA; [b] Frances Payne Bolton School of Nursing at Case Western Reserve University, Health Education Campus, 10900 Euclid Avenue, Cleveland, OH 44106-7343, USA; [c] School of Dental Medicine at Case Western Reserve University, Health Education Campus, 10900 Euclid Avenue, Cleveland, OH 44106-7343, USA
* Corresponding author.
E-mail address: mildac@uw.edu

Dent Clin N Am 67 (2023) 707–709
https://doi.org/10.1016/j.cden.2023.05.029
0011-8532/23/

DENTAL MANAGEMENT DECISION AND JUSTIFICATION

Gestational diabetes mellitus (GDM) is a temporary condition in which women who have not previously had diabetes develop elevated blood sugars during pregnancy. Screening is recommended for all pregnant women after 24 weeks of gestation. Diagnosis is made by completing an oral glucose tolerance test that consists of patients consuming a large amount of sugar (a glucose challenge) and testing the point glucose 2 hours later.[1] Hemoglobin A1c is not useful for diagnosis or assessing control in GDM due to changes in hemoglobin levels during pregnancy.[2] Instead, dentists can gauge the level of glycemic control by asking the patient what the blood sugar levels have been over the last 2 weeks. **Table 1** lists target glucose levels in women with GDM.

The management of gestational diabetes starts with dietary modifications, physical exercise, and self-glucose monitoring. However, if individuals are not able to reach the target glycemic levels, medications may be appropriate. Individuals who have gestational diabetes have an increased risk of developing type II diabetes in the future and are recommended to be screened 12 weeks post partum as well as every 3 years.[1]

Women should be counselled on the importance of maintaining oral health throughout their pregnancy. Although there is insufficient evidence that treatment of periodontal disease will prevent or improve adverse pregnancy outcomes such as preterm birth or preeclampsia, it can improve maternal oral health and is not associated with any adverse outcomes.[3] In addition, improved maternal oral health can limit the spread of cariogenic bacteria to off-spring, decreasing the risk of early childhood caries. A national consensus statement represented by the American College of Obstetricians and Gynecologists and the American Dental Association encourages prenatal health care professionals and dental professionals to work together in identifying, referring, and treating oral disease in pregnant patients.[4] Management of pregnant patients with gestational diabetes should follow general principles of dental management in pregnant patients as well as those with diabetes. In this case, it is appropriate to order and take the radiographs needed using a lead apron and thyroid collar and scale and root planing of the teeth. Local anesthesia with vasoconstrictors is safe to use as long as the recommended dose is not exceeded. If the patient's blood sugar levels have been within the recommended range no increased risk of postoperative complications is anticipated. When individuals report multiple blood sugar readings outside the recommended range (see **Table 1**) they should be referred to their obstetrician for further evaluation and management and one may consider to delay nonemergency dental treatment if the risk of infection or poor wound healing outweighs the benefits of the planned procedure. If analgesics are required after the procedure, acetaminophen is preferred, and the patient's obstetrician can be consulted. Patients with elevated blood pressure should be referred to a physician, as it could be a sign of

Table 1
Target glucose values in women with gestational diabetes mellitus

Timing	Target Glucose Values
Fasting	$\leq$ 95 mg/dL (5.3 mmol/L)
One-h postprandial	$\leq$ 140 mg/dL (7.8 mmol/L)
Two-h postprandial	$\leq$ 120 mg/dL (6.7 mmol/L)

Created from Resource 1.

preeclampsia.[5] Patients who are pregnant and/or have gestational diabetes can be safely treated in outpatient dental clinics when appropriate patient assessment and management are applied.

CLINICS CARE POINTS

- Hemoglobin A1c is not useful for diagnosis or assessing control in GDM due to changes in hemoglobin levels during pregnancy.
- Assessing blood sugar levels over the last 2 weeks can help gauge the level of glycemic control in patients with GDM.
- Providing dental care during pregnancy is not associated with any adverse outcomes and maintaining oral health throughout pregnancy is recommended.

REFERENCES

1. Garrison A. Screening, diagnosis, and management of gestational diabetes mellitus. Am Fam Physician 2015;91(7):460–7.
2. Edelson PK, James KE, Leong A, et al. Longitudinal changes in the relationship between hemoglobin A1c and glucose tolerance across pregnancy and postpartum. J Clin Endocrinol Metab 2020;105(5):e1999–2007.
3. Newnham JP, Newnham IA, Ball C MI, et al. Treatment of periodontal disease during pregnancy: a randomized controlled trial. Obstet Gynecol 2009;114(6):1239–48.
4. Oral Health Care During Pregnancy Expert Workgroup. Oral health care during pregnancy: a national consensus statement. Washington, DC: National Maternal and Child Oral Health Resource Center; 2012.
5. Little J, Miller C, Rhodus N. Diabetes *in* little and falace's dental management of the medically compromised patient. Ninth ed. St. Louis, Missouri: Eslevier; 2018. Available at: http://ezsecureaccess.balamand.edu.lb/login?url=https://www.clinicalkey.com/dura/browse/bookChapter/3-s2.0-C20150014228. Accessed September 20, 2022.

procedures. Patients who are pregnant and/or have gestational diabetes can be safely treated in outpatient dental clinics when appropriate patient assessment and management are applied.

[illegible]

[illegible]

REFERENCES

[illegible]

Restorative Dental Treatment and Endodontic Surgery in a Pregnant Patient Receiving Corticosteroids

Fatmah Alhendi, BMedSc, DDS, MSOB

KEYWORDS

• Corticosteroids • Pregnancy • Odontology • Management • Adrenal insufficiency

KEY POINTS

- Corticosteroid therapy (CST) is common in pregnancy to treat recurrent miscarriages or fetal abnormalities.
- Elective dental procedures in pregnancy are preferred to be carried out in the second trimester.
- Long-term use of corticosteroids can lead to adrenal suppression, immunosuppression, Cushing syndrome, hyperglycemia, osteoporosis, hypertension, and peptic ulcer among other.
- The risk of adrenal crisis at the dental clinic due to use of exogenous corticosteroids depends on the dosage, duration of treatment, route of administration, frequency, time lapse since the last dose, and type of procedure performed.
- Current evidence found that patients on corticosteroid therapy undergoing general dental procedures or minor surgical procedures under local anesthesia do not require supplementary corticosteroids and should only maintain their regular dose of corticosteroids.

MEDICAL SCENARIO

A 29-year-old pregnant woman at the beginning of her third trimester presented to the dental clinic for restoration of a painful carious upper premolar tooth and a possible endodontic surgery for a previously root canal–treated lower molar tooth that is recurrently getting infected. During history taking, the patient reported that she is on a single weekly dose of 11.4 milligrams of betamethasone therapy for up to 32 weeks' gestation as antenatal steroid (ANS) for an anticipation of a preterm birth.

DENTAL MANAGEMENT DECISION AND JUSTIFICATION

The use of ANS therapy is common and is the standard care for pregnant women with risk of recurrent miscarriages, fetal abnormalities, or premature delivery due to its

Ministry of Health, AlSulaibikhat, Jamal Abdulnasser Street, PO Box 5, Zip Code 13001, Kuwait
E-mail address: falhendi@alumni.upenn.edu

Dent Clin N Am 67 (2023) 711–712
https://doi.org/10.1016/j.cden.2023.05.030
dental.theclinics.com

effect on the maturation of fetal pulmonary function.[1] Long-term CST can result in secondary adrenal insufficiency due to its effect on the hypothalamic-pituitary-adrenal axis and the resulting suppression of the endogenous cortisol level that is used to maintain homeostasis.[2] In addition to the adrenal suppression, several adverse effect can appear with long-term CST such as immunosuppression, Cushing syndrome, hyperglycemia, osteoporosis, hypertension, and peptic ulcer among others.[2] Adrenal insufficiency can be primary, caused by disease of the adrenal cortex, or secondary, such as in the use of exogenous CST.[2] Recent evidence suggests that only patients with primary adrenal insufficiency may need to receive supplementary CST before major surgeries under general anesthesia, whereas patient with secondary adrenal insufficiency receiving any dental or minor surgical procedure, like in our case scenario, needs only their regular corticosteroid dose before the surgical procedure.[3] In the case of complex surgical procedure under general anesthesia, patient physician should be consulted regarding preoperative corticosteroid supplementation, as it depends on the complexity of the procedure and the preexisting corticosteroid dose.[4] Because long-term CST can elevate blood pressure and blood glucose level, preoperative measurement of both should be carried out.[4] In our case, the patient was in pain and the dental treatment cannot be postponed till the end of pregnancy. Lidocaine 2% with epinephrine as a local anesthetic agent can be safely administered for the patient, and the postoperative pain can be managed with acetaminophen as the drug of choice to control pain during pregnancy.[5]

CLINICAL CARE POINTS

- The use of corticosteroid therapy is not uncommon in complicated pregnancies.
- Long-term corticosteroids intake is linked to many serious medical conditions, such as adrenal crisis, that can complicate dental treatment.
- As a general rule , patients on corticosteroid therapy undergoing general dental procedures under local anaesthesia do not require supplementary corticosteroids.

FINANCIAL SUPPORT AND SPONSORSHIP

Nil.

CONFLICTS OF INTEREST

There are no conflicts of interest.

REFERENCES

1. Kemp MW, Newnham JP, Challis JG, et al. The clinical use of corticosteroids in pregnancy. Hum Reprod Update 2016;22(2):240–59.
2. Hargitai L, Sherman CR. Corticosteroids in dentistry. Clin Update 2001;23:11–2.
3. Marik PE, Varon J. Requirement of perioperative stress doses of corticosteroids: a systematic review of the literature. Arch Surg 2008;143(12):1222–6.
4. Gibson N, Ferguson JW. Steroid cover for dental patients on long-term steroid medication: proposed clinical guidelines based upon a critical review of the literature. Br Dent J 2004;197(11):681–5.
5. Little JW, Miller C, Rhodus NL. Dental management of the medically compromised patient - E-book on VitalSource. 9th edition. Elsevier Health Sciences; 2017.

UNITED STATES POSTAL SERVICE®

Statement of Ownership, Management, and Circulation (All Periodicals Publications Except Requester Publications)

1. Publication Title: DENTAL CLINICS OF NORTH AMERICA	2. Publication Number: 566 – 480	3. Filing Date: 9/18/2023
4. Issue Frequency: JAN, APR, JUL, OCT	5. Number of Issues Published Annually: 4	6. Annual Subscription Price: $333.00

7. Complete Mailing Address of Known Office of Publication *(Not printer) (Street, city, county, state, and ZIP+4®)*
ELSEVIER INC.
230 Park Avenue, Suite 800
New York, NY 10169

Contact Person: Malathi Samayan
Telephone *(Include area code)*: 91-44-4299-4507

8. Complete Mailing Address of Headquarters or General Business Office of Publisher *(Not printer)*
ELSEVIER INC.
230 Park Avenue, Suite 800
New York, NY 10169

9. Full Names and Complete Mailing Addresses of Publisher, Editor, and Managing Editor *(Do not leave blank)*

Publisher *(Name and complete mailing address)*
Dolores Meloni, ELSEVIER INC.
1600 JOHN F KENNEDY BLVD. SUITE 1600
PHILADELPHIA, PA 19103-2899

Editor *(Name and complete mailing address)*
JOHN VASSALLO, ELSEVIER INC.
1600 JOHN F KENNEDY BLVD. SUITE 1600
PHILADELPHIA, PA 19103-2899

Managing Editor *(Name and complete mailing address)*
PATRICK MANLEY, ELSEVIER INC.
1600 JOHN F KENNEDY BLVD. SUITE 1600
PHILADELPHIA, PA 19103-2899

10. Owner *(Do not leave blank. If the publication is owned by a corporation, give the name and address of the corporation immediately followed by the names and addresses of all stockholders owning or holding 1 percent or more of the total amount of stock. If not owned by a corporation, give the names and addresses of the individual owners. If owned by a partnership or other unincorporated firm, give its name and address as well as those of each individual owner. If the publication is published by a nonprofit organization, give its name and address.)*

Full Name	Complete Mailing Address
WHOLLY OWNED SUBSIDIARY OF REED/ELSEVIER, US HOLDINGS	1600 JOHN F KENNEDY BLVD. SUITE 1600 PHILADELPHIA, PA 19103-2899

11. Known Bondholders, Mortgagees, and Other Security Holders Owning or Holding 1 Percent or More of Total Amount of Bonds, Mortgages, or Other Securities. If none, check box → ☐ None

Full Name	Complete Mailing Address
N/A	

12. Tax Status *(For completion by nonprofit organizations authorized to mail at nonprofit rates) (Check one)*
The purpose, function, and nonprofit status of this organization and the exempt status for federal income tax purposes:
☒ Has Not Changed During Preceding 12 Months
☐ Has Changed During Preceding 12 Months *(Publisher must submit explanation of change with this statement)*

13. Publication Title: DENTAL CLINICS OF NORTH AMERICA
14. Issue Date for Circulation Data Below: JULY 2023

15. Extent and Nature of Circulation			Average No. Copies Each Issue During Preceding 12 Months	No. Copies of Single Issue Published Nearest to Filing Date
a. Total Number of Copies *(Net press run)*			167	136
b. Paid Circulation *(By Mail and Outside the Mail)*	(1)	Mailed Outside-County Paid Subscriptions Stated on PS Form 3541 (Include paid distribution above nominal rate, advertiser's proof copies, and exchange copies)	90	70
	(2)	Mailed In-County Paid Subscriptions Stated on PS Form 3541 *(Include paid distribution above nominal rate, advertiser's proof copies, and exchange copies)*	0	0
	(3)	Paid Distribution Outside the Mails Including Sales Through Dealers and Carriers, Street Vendors, Counter Sales, and Other Paid Distribution Outside USPS®	50	43
	(4)	Paid Distribution by Other Classes of Mail Through the USPS (e.g., First-Class Mail®)	24	20
c. Total Paid Distribution *[Sum of 15b (1), (2), (3), and (4)]*			164	133
d. Free or Nominal Rate Distribution *(By Mail and Outside the Mail)*	(1)	Free or Nominal Rate Outside-County Copies included on PS Form 3541	2	2
	(2)	Free or Nominal Rate In-County Copies Included on PS Form 3541	0	0
	(3)	Free or Nominal Rate Copies Mailed at Other Classes Through the USPS (e.g., First-Class Mail)	0	0
	(4)	Free or Nominal Rate Distribution Outside the Mail *(Carriers or other means)*	1	1
e. Total Free or Nominal Rate Distribution *(Sum of 15d (1), (2), (3) and (4))*			3	3
f. Total Distribution *(Sum of 15c and 15e)*			167	136
g. Copies not Distributed *(See Instructions to Publishers #4 (page #3))*			0	0
h. Total *(Sum of 15f and g)*			167	136
i. Percent Paid *(15c divided by 15f times 100)*			98.5%	97.79%

* If you are claiming electronic copies, go to line 16 on page 3. If you are not claiming electronic copies, skip to line 17 on page 3.

16. Electronic Copy Circulation	Average No. Copies Each Issue During Preceding 12 Months	No. Copies of Single Issue Published Nearest to Filing Date
a. Paid Electronic Copies		
b. Total Paid Print Copies (Line 15c) + Paid Electronic Copies (Line 16a)		
c. Total Print Distribution (Line 15f) + Paid Electronic Copies (Line 16a)		
d. Percent Paid (Both Print & Electronic Copies) (16b divided by 16c × 100)		

☒ **I certify that 50% of all my distributed copies (electronic and print) are paid above a nominal price.**

17. Publication of Statement of Ownership
☒ If the publication is a general publication, publication of this statement is required. Will be printed in the OCTOBER 2023 issue of this publication. ☐ Publication not required.

18. Signature and Title of Editor, Publisher, Business Manager, or Owner
Malathi Samayan - Distribution Controller — *Malathi Samayan* — Date: 9/18/2023

I certify that all information furnished on this form is true and complete. I understand that anyone who furnishes false or misleading information on this form or who omits material or information requested on the form may be subject to criminal sanctions (including fines and imprisonment) and/or civil sanctions (including civil penalties).

Printed and bound by CPI Group (UK) Ltd, Croydon, CR0 4YY
03/10/2024
01040466-0014